'An important contribution at an important time... Martinus explores the unique challenges faced by teens and how yoga offers a valuable wellbeing toolbox to live an optimal life. Covering essential topics from depression to addiction, this book offers simple, practical, tried-and-tested techniques. For those teaching teens, this is essential reading.'

– *Simon Haas, teacher of yoga philosophy and author of* The Book of Dharma *and* Yoga and the Dark Night of the Soul

'Charlotta Martinus brings out the challenges and opportunities facing teenagers today and shows how yoga is a solution and a way to optimize their potential. In a rapidly changing world teenagers everywhere are vulnerable, yet receptive to practices like yoga; this is highlighted with interesting anecdotes, information and empathy for the problems faced by young people. The book skilfully blends theory and practice, and all yoga therapists, teachers and parents would benefit from reading it.'

– *Shirley Telles, MBBS, PhD (Neurophysiology), Director, Pantanjali Research Foundation, India*

'Recent research documents that yoga can promote mental health and wellbeing. Adolescence can be a rather stressful period of life, so yoga is likely to be especially relevant for teens. Charlotta Martinus is a world-leading expert on yoga for teens, and this book targets yoga teachers, yoga therapists, teenagers and parents. I expect that they will welcome this book as much as I do.'

– *Ingunn Hagen, Professor, Department of Psychology, Norwegian University of Science and Technology (NTNU)*

'While I was overseeing police youth strategy in Somerset I witnessed how the 'Teen Yoga' programme was consistently able to help and guide young people to become well-rounded, grounded, thoughtful and compassionate citizens. I saw how it addressed existing angst, heartache and behavioural issues in young people who were struggling to understand their lives and emotions. I cannot recommend this guide to those and supporting young people enough.

This comprehensive, easy-to-read, structured and evidenced guide is a must-have for those working in youth development, mental health or simply working with common teen issues.'

– *Dr Simon Selby, PhD, PGCE, CLJ, Visiting Lecturer in Criminal Justice*

'As an educator, mental health professional and yoga therapist working with teens, this is the book that so many of us have been waiting for.

Charlotta brings forth a well-balanced mixture of the evidence base, experience and opportunity for personal engagement and reflections on the work. She offers many practices and exercises to share with young people and to deepen our own practice in an accessible and informative way.'

– *Dr Lucy Arnsby-Wilson, clinical psychologist, Director and Founder of The Maya Project*

'The ancient practice of yoga is hugely relevant today. This book sets out the theoretical underpinnings and promising emerging evidence base for the benefits of yoga for adolescents. With a host of practical techniques and tips, Charlotta shares her insight and experience of teaching yoga to teenagers. This book is essential reading for yoga teachers working with teenagers and an important contribution to the wider agenda of increasing the reach of this holistic practice.'

– *Dr Vaishnavee Madden, Consultant in Public Health, UK*

TEEN YOGA FOR YOGA THERAPISTS

of related interest

Yoga Therapy for Fear
Treating Anxiety, Depression and Rage with the Vagus Nerve and Other Techniques
Beth Spindler with Kat Heagberg and Kevin Richardson
ISBN 978 1 84819 374 1
eISBN 978 0 85701 331 6

Principles and Themes in Yoga Therapy
An Introduction to Integrative Mind/Body Yoga Therapeutics
James Foulkes
Foreword by Mikhail Kogan, MD
Illustrated by Simon Barkworth
ISBN 978 1 84819 248 5
eISBN 978 0 85701 194 7

Trauma-Sensitive Yoga
Dagmar Härle
Foreword by David Emerson
ISBN 978 1 84819 346 8
eISBN 978 0 85701 301 9

Ocean of Yoga
Meditations on Yoga and Ayurveda for Balance, Awareness, and Well-Being
Julie Dunlop
Foreword by Vasant Lad
ISBN 978 1 84819 360 4
eISBN 978 0 85701 318 7

TEEN YOGA FOR YOGA THERAPISTS

A Guide to Development, Mental Health and Working with Common Teen Issues

CHARLOTTA MARTINUS

Foreword by Sir Anthony Seldon

Graphics by Sofia Kearney

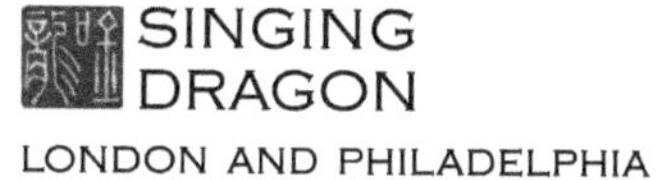

LONDON AND PHILADELPHIA

'You can be the person that you like to be in yoga' poster reproduced here with kind permission from Amy Morgan, Institute of Psychological Sciences, University of Leeds.

First published in 2018
by Singing Dragon
an imprint of Jessica Kingsley Publishers
73 Collier Street
London N1 9BE, UK
and
400 Market Street, Suite 400
Philadelphia, PA 19106, USA

www.singingdragon.com

Front cover image source: Pexels. The cover image is for illustrative purposes only, and any person featuring is a model.

Library of Congress Cataloging in Publication Data
Names: Martinus, Charlotta, author.
Title: Teen yoga for yoga therapists : a guide to development, mental health and working with common teen issues / Charlotta Martinus ; foreword by Sir Anthony Seldon.
Description: London ; Philadelphia : Jessica Kingsley Publishers, 2018. | Includes bibliographical references and index.
Identifiers: LCCN 2018007490 | ISBN 9781848193994 (alk. paper)
Subjects: | MESH: Yoga--psychology | Psychology, Adolescent | Adolescent Psychiatry--methods | Mindfulness
Classification: LCC RA781.7 | NLM WS 462 | DDC 613.7/0460835--
dc23 LC record available at https://lccn.loc.gov/2018007490

British Library Cataloguing in Publication Data
A CIP catalogue record for this book is available from the British Library

ISBN 978 1 84819 399 4
eISBN 978 0 85701 355 2

Printed and bound in Great Britain

Contents

Part III

Foreword

I'm very pleased indeed to be writing the foreword for this book. I did not start yoga and meditation until I was 25 and have practised ever since. They have changed my life and thinking utterly for the better and I keep thinking how much better it would have been had I started earlier.

There are three reasons why I strongly support yoga and meditation for young people. First, they are natural. Yoga goes with the brain of the body, and it helps all of us to breathe properly, exercise properly, sleep well and relax deeply. Yoga works by helping the body to work naturally and well. Meditation achieves the same for the mind. It helps the mind to work naturally at its best.

Second, we now know from ample well-evidenced studies that habits that are learned when young remain with us for much longer. If people can experience the physical, mental and emotional benefits of yoga and meditation when they are still young, they will have acquired habits for a lifetime. I believe that they will turn to alcohol and drugs less when the difficult times come, and they will be able to cope better because their minds and their bodies have become more resilient and better able to cope with the difficulties, sadnesses and stresses that life throws at us all.

Third, and finally, yoga and meditation help slow us down in a world where we are being made to move at ever faster speeds, and where the mental health of young people, partly as a result, is deteriorating at an alarming rate. Yoga and meditation will help our young people to slow down and cope better. Much more than this, though, it will help them to live life to the full, to enjoy their relationships, nature, their work, the arts and indeed all of life much more to the full.

I strongly endorse the approach that this volume advocates, and believe that the young people lucky enough to follow it will gain immeasurably as a result.

Sir Anthony Seldon, FRSA, FRHistS, FKC
Chancellor of the University of Buckingham
June 2018

Acknowledgements

Thank you to my sons Adam and Alex, who started me on this path and have guided me every step of the way. My partner Nick has had the unenviable job of editing my enthusiastic ramblings and has continuously picked me up out of many moments of despondency, when the topic of this book has simply seemed too big and complicated to master. My mum, who has written and published many books herself, mentioned to me as a teenager that I should write and has given me so much confidence in myself, my power and my voice. As a teacher, my mum lit the flame of compassion for young people in me, when I was one myself, through her own years of dedication to teens. My dad, who continuously surprised me with his unfathomable confidence in my ability to take on the world and who is with me every day in spirit. All my countless teachers have guided me selflessly over the years and ultimately my yoga teachers and masters who opened my eyes to the truth, Swami Sivananda, Swami Vishnu-Devananda and Swami Govindananda.

I would like to acknowledge the support and guidance of Dr Sat Bir Khalsa and Dr Shirley Telles who have become colleagues on the journey of yoga and young people. Their tireless work in the field of research is astounding and inspiring. I would also like to acknowledge the powerful and clear contribution of Simon Haas who has made yoga philosophy so easy for my students to access through his work *The Dharma Code*. Dr Siegel remains my touchstone when it comes to understanding the adolescent brain and the impact of yoga and mindfulness on the brain function of a teenager. Thanks, Dan, also for your lecture on the TeenYoga course. Dr Mel Wood, paediatric neurologist and trainee psychiatrist in child and adolescent mental health services (CAMHS), has contributed to Chapter 3. The Kripalu Institute in

Massachusetts set me off on the journey of writing this book, after we attended their excellent Yoga in Schools symposium in 2016. Vic Williams took many hours to read, comment and feed back on the first renditions of the book in 2016 and 2017, which was hugely helpful and encouraging. I would also like to acknowledge the support of all the students who come on the TeenYoga course and have contributed to my understanding more than they will ever know. Keep coming together at the Instill Conference every year in London, so that we can continue to inspire each other! There are countless others who do not wish to be acknowledged who I would like to thank for their concrete contributions in their special fields. Lastly, I would like to acknowledge the immense impact that head teachers, teachers, teaching assistants and pupils have had in encouraging yoga in their schools.

Preface

Fatima had fed her nephew supper and finished bathing her niece, she shut the door, took off her shela, her abhaya, and rolled out her mat. As she started to relax on the mat, the day seeped out of her bones and into the ground below. The arguments at college, the mother's expectations, the niece, the nephews and the unwelcome gaze. As she started her movements, the sensations in the body rose to the fore, tensions reaching their peak and then releasing, sometimes with a tear rolling down her cheek, with the diffuse memory of discomfort, shame or confusion. With each posture, she was reclaiming her body, becoming powerful again. With compassion and awareness, she watched her sensations, feelings, emotions and thoughts as they emerged and allowed the pain, the suffering, the joy to travel through her body in the practice, offering it all up to the universe, or into the mat. The disparate parts of her body started to feel as one, fluid and connected. Her mind diffused into the body, no longer separate, ruminating. Grounding herself, reclaiming her body, her mind became calm. Coming to the end of her practice she connected with her breath, witnessing the echo of the sensations travelling around her body and her mind let go of haunting visions of improper touch. Coming into stillness, coming into forgiveness, travelling through the pain again and again. As she dropped into relaxation on her mat, safe and supported, she knew that, in that moment, nothing was required of her, she was good enough. The anger had dissipated and, in its place, she felt a deep sense of peace within her body and mind, a connection to herself and those around her once more. I am home, I have arrived home. (A story from one of the students I teach, who wishes to remain anonymous, and agreed that yoga had helped her inhabit her faith more authentically and overcome abuse)

I imagine that the alarming issues prevalent among young people today propel you to read this book and me to write it. We come together in a field, where yoga takes its rightful place as a potential lifestyle choice, at a time where the young person is looking for the third guru, the teacher. The mother is the first guru, from birth to the first 'big' tooth at 7, the father is the second guru, from the first adult tooth to menarche or spermarche at around 14, and the teacher as guru (remover of darkness) is the third guru from 14 to around 21 in traditional yoga culture. Yoga has been my guru, through my own practice (daily meditation for 20 years), the ancient texts and my own teachers. Like so many others who come on my courses I say, if only I had come across yoga as a teen I would have made better choices and my life would have turned out very differently.

When yoga found me at the mature age of 33, I felt that my world somehow rearranged itself, values fell into place, other values dropped away, new friends appeared and old ones phased out, new optimal habits took root and other destructive ones melted away, effortlessly. My confidence and courage shot through the roof. I belonged to a non-judgemental, supportive, clearly boundaried context – my yoga *shala*. The London Sivananda Centre was a refuge for thousands of us, who found sanity in a mad world. Lifelong relationships still have their genesis at this centre under the infinitely compassionate guidance and gaze of teachers and swamis, who continuously help us to bring our life experiences into the context of yoga with weekly philosophy lectures and meditation sessions. It became, and still is, my spiritual home. Still today, we are all, metaphorically speaking, walking each other home (checking in with each other, helping each other out, supporting and contributing to each other's yoga journeys all over the world). Often my students refer to me as their spiritual mother and I feel the same enormous tenderness towards them, as if they were my children. Similarly, my colleagues and friends from the Sivananda Centre genuinely feel like my sisters and brothers.

This book is the result of 30 years of experience working with either young people or yoga, or both combined. It has also been shaped and inspired by my 15 years as a single mother of two beautiful young men. I have been invited to teach and humbly witnessed the flowering of yoga in many varied contexts, from the slums of Sierra Leone, through urban drug addiction centres, to traditional Arab Muslim groups in Abu Dhabi, to supporting those with suicidal ideation, to homeless London teenagers, to energetic, joyful and well-adapted teens who are curious and keen to adopt alternative lifestyle choices.

When we soften the heart and live in compassion, it is impossible to ignore suffering. It was obvious to me that I would bring the yoga that had supported me in such a fundamental way to children who are looking for guidance. Yoga creates a matrix by which to live, guiding every area of our lives, through enhanced intuition, guided by the first law – love (*ahimsa*), compassion, non-harming.

Since my lifestyle and quality of life have improved so fundamentally due to yoga, it feels important to share these profound teachings with other practitioners who seem to hold a narrower view of the potential and practice of yoga. As yoga becomes more popular, it is becoming increasingly fragmented, in most contexts focusing more on physical benefits and ignoring our emotional, mental, spiritual and social dimensions. Yoga means union, connection, coming together. If we are separating our body from our mind or any other aspect of being human, we are not moving towards unity but towards dissolution, fragmentation and isolation. This book aims, in some small way, to rectify this misunderstanding of yoga and create an offering for our young people and the reader, which invites them and you to dive deeply into this human experience and create optimistic and healthy futures for themselves and our planet. With your help I believe we can help them build a more peaceful and unified world.

INTRODUCTION

I have always really enjoyed spending time with teenagers. As a modern foreign language teacher in the 1980s and 1990s, I was told that I was particularly good at engaging and sharing my knowledge in an entertaining and interesting way. I took a break for a few years and returned in 2003 to a very different world. My friend and colleague asked if I could cover her yoga classes at the local secondary school in Somerset while she went to Australia. I was shocked. Stress levels had risen to a degree that was affecting focus, discipline and academic performance. Boys and girls were obsessed by their looks and what others thought of them and seemed much more fragile than before. Boys were hitting each other over the heads with the yoga mats, rolling in them, making 'sausage rolls', jeering at the girls' bottoms in front of them and the girls were focused on my 'camel toe' – I had to look up the word! I came out utterly dejected. It was a disappointing and disillusioning experience – teaching teens yoga today was a completely different ball game from teaching them French all those years ago and vastly different from teaching little children or adults. A new universe. I had to re-evaluate the whole rationale and methodology of sharing yoga.

When do you come across teens in your daily life? Across the kitchen table? On the bus? In the shopping mall? In the pub? How do you feel about them? How much do you know about what goes on behind that perfectly made-up mask – can you see the persona?

Take a moment here to journal your responses.

How to read this book

To make this book useful to you, I am drawing on the broad and deep tradition of integral yoga. The lineage, as do so many from

India, accentuates the importance of all aspects of yoga, including postures, breathing practice, meditation, mindfulness, relaxation, *nidra*[1] and visualisation, to name but a few. At times I will invite you to reflect and maybe write some ideas in a book. You might like to keep a journal to keep track of your impressions, intentions and ideas.

I would ask you to imagine a hypothetical group in front of you (define whether they want to be there or not, whether the group is mixed or single gender, what age they are and so on) and ask yourself: which aspect of yoga do we best apply to this particular situation? How do I serve this group in the best possible way? How do I meet them where they are? As most of us are aware, a group has many individuals with different needs but there is also a group dynamic, which can be sensed at any time. Feeling into the dynamic of the group and, to some extent, the individual needs of the group, you may ask yourself the following question: How can I reach this teen in the best possible way, so they feel seen and heard by me and so their deepest needs are met by the science I embody?

Take a moment to reflect on these questions.

Part I of the book is an exploration of some major aspects of being young today, giving you I hope some context in which to understand their lives. I delve through the different layers of perception, starting with the brain and ending with spirituality. Part II deals with practices to support young people in typical situations which you may encounter. Part III explores spirituality and optimal wellness.

In 2008 CAMHS noted that 'Anyone working directly with children and families needs to ask themselves regularly "what can I do to improve the mental health and well-being of this child?"'[2] The need for some kind of holistic approach to health among teens is clearly so necessary and yet so lacking. I hope in this book to throw some light on how yoga might support optimal wellness for young people.

The courses I have been running since 2004 (around 200 students a year) involve rich conversations between professionals from different fields, reflecting on current situations in their

---

1 *Nidra*, which means sleep in Sanskrit, is a relaxation exercise practised by scanning the body and relaxing each part in turn.

2 Department of Health 2008.

area, whether medicine, education or therapy. They are a time for deep reflection and signposting to further reading, reflection or courses, in order to find our true dharma. We all learn so much in this format. I will try to distil some of these beautiful conversations here.

Background

In the last ten years, obesity among young people has doubled. In the UK today 1 in 4 young people (aged 13–17) has a diagnosable mental health issue; young people are the biggest group to access the NHS after old people. Osteoporosis, rheumatoid arthritis, depression, self-harm, addiction, sleep deprivation and suicide among young men have all been rising in most areas of the UK over the past few years according to reports by YoungMinds and the NSPCC.[3]

When asked at the recent Instill Conference (the annual Teen Yoga Foundation conference for Yoga, Education and Research) in London, young people spoke with one voice, saying 'we are aware of the mental health issues but give us tools to deal with them!'[4]

The information is out there, schools have counsellors and have been asked to appoint a mental health lead in every institution. Young people realise that they are struggling, and they are asking for tools. Medication for many is the last step; they are actively looking for other ways to cope with an increasingly stressful world. Some find solace on the internet, others in the family, others in friendship, but most either self-medicate with illegal or prescribed drugs or they struggle in silence.

Learning how to share yoga

After being shocked into urgent reflection, my next steps were focused on learning how to reach young people with one of the most precious toolkits I had ever come across, namely yoga. I set about chatting with them one to one or in groups after class, I made notes, spoke to their tutors, sat around in the staffroom to find

3 YoungMinds 2018; NSPCC 2018.
4 Cross 2017.

out the atmosphere there and feel into the morale of the teachers. I researched education policy and looked at recent psychological papers. I took on more and more groups in various schools. I took a 350-hour yoga therapy for mental health course and I reached out to my own teachers and reflected and wrote notes. I started working as a yoga therapist for CAMHS, working at a sectioned unit for those struggling with mental health issues. Each week, over a period of two years, I tried something new, something different, I broadened my understanding of yoga, I delved deep into the Vedic texts. I changed the groups, making some gender specific, making them smaller, bringing in teacher assistants, until we got the 'recipe' right. I tried and tested the recipe in different circumstances, in different schools, until I was completely satisfied. Some of what I learned over the past 14 years of teaching yoga and 30 years of teaching in general, in response to the needs of today's youth, is here, for you to use, so I hope you will be better equipped than I was! My hard work and insistence in sharing this practice with young people all over the world and with more than 700 teachers (reaching tens of thousands of students) in over 20 countries has always been rewarding as I reflect on how I have managed to apply yoga to every conceivable community, from the child soldiers of Sierra Leone to Abu Dhabi sheikhs, through to schools in Tobago.

One of the most delightful testimonies to TeenYoga was on a course, when we were sharing our reasons for coming, and one student paused and looked me gently in the eyes for what felt like a long time and, finally, said, 'Do you remember me? You taught me when I was 14; since then I have wanted to do what you do, and I am now 24 and teaching yoga at my school.' My heart skipped a beat as I welled with emotion, the others in the room gasped and time stood still as I remembered her vividly, eyes fixed on me and my every move, ten years ago.

I guess the main questions for me were always, what is yoga, why yoga for these young people – how is this ancient science relevant? Why would they be interested? Maybe you would like to reflect on this before you go further.

PART I

— Chapter 1 —

WHAT IS YOGA?

Taken in its entirety, yoga functions as a complete, holistic and continuous healing modality, which encompasses all elements of being human – appealing to physical, mental, emotional, community and spiritual needs of our being. In my view, this holistic approach is its strength and power.

Radical self-care

As prominent researcher in yoga for young people, Professor Sat Bir Khalsa, says, yoga supports 'global functionality' through its ability to promote meta-cognition.[1] (Meta-cognition is when we are able to have an overview of our own experience, whether physical, mental or emotional, and understand it in the context of others and our global functionality.)

Adapt, adjust, accommodate, do good, be good – these axioms are emblazoned in my mind as being at the core of yoga. They were written up on the walls of the first ever ashram I visited in India back in 2000: the Neyyar Dam Ashram in Kerala, southern India, which is devoted to the great yoga master Swami Sivananda and his disciple who brought yoga to the West, Swami Vishnu-Devananda.

When we are able to allow others to live their lives without judgement, without trying to control or organise them, our community can live in peace and harmony. Being 'good' might be an old-fashioned concept. But the idea of lifting myself above the regular flood of impressions that pass unexamined into my mind and memory, choosing compassion over judgement and connection over antagonism, will inevitably create yoga – union.

1 Khalsa 2016.

The clear understanding that by caring for myself I will become expert at caring for others was always my understanding from the texts. *Yogas Chitta Vritti Nirodhah* (Yoga is the Stilling of the Mind Waves) outlines this perfectly.[2] The quality of relationship I have with myself determines completely the quality of relationship I might have with another (this is not an unusual idea, completely supported by modern psychologists and philosophers). The degree to which we manage to rest in the peace of our minds relates directly to the impact we will have on others around us, the peace we are able to emanate and ultimately to world peace. If the 'yoga' we are practising is not eliciting peace, then it is not creating union within our selves, then by definition it cannot be yoga.

Many students on my courses have completed a full teacher training course and have been practising for decades, yet they lack fundamental understanding of the breadth of yoga. I know that many yoga teacher training courses that are being offered at the moment are more in favour of the physical practice at the expense of the philosophy and core of yoga. These teachers and therapists are then not able to access or share the deep and more useful aspects of yoga, which would be of greater help to young people. I hope to be able to support a more in-depth understanding and guide the reader to various rich yoga practices that could enhance the lives of young people.

In this book I will attempt to present yoga in a way that I truly believe could have a massive impact on mental health. At its very core are the full gamut of practices that bring us to that complete experience. These practices are commonly known as the eight limbs of yoga.

Shift in perspective

Asana forms a large part of what we see yoga to be, and certainly for your students, the teens, it will be the main image of yoga – the Instagram sylphs in fashionable lycra performing extraordinary physical feats. However, over the past 13 years that I have been working with young people, there has been a shift in perspective

---

2 Durgananda 2010.

from 'Miss, can you do the splits?' to 'I've come to yoga because I can't sleep at night.'

This shift is fundamental and intrinsic. As we move forward, deepening our true understanding of yoga, we are able to honour it in its true majesty. The attraction of yoga today lies in the very fact that it is a holistic science, that thoroughly addresses every part of being human. Herein lies the success of true yoga and it is where pilates, dance and pure asana by itself fall short. With mindfulness initiatives, we see a focus on mental health, by itself, as if we were divorced from our body in that moment. In an asana class we are not necessarily tuning into the state of mind but may instead be distracting ourselves with physical activity. At church, temple or mosque, we focus on our spiritual needs without necessarily acknowledging that we have a physical body or mind!

With this disjointed, disconnected and fragmented view of human experience and existence, no wonder there is a feeling of dis-ease and isolation. We are literally isolating each part of ourselves from the other just as we isolate each one of us from the other. However, yoga teaches us that we are one – we are one with our body, mind and soul, we are one with our family, we are one with our society and one with our world and universe. This is the teaching of yoga and the teaching of om.[3]

When we deliver a whole person approach we are bringing the individual to peace and balance. This is also why we advocate a whole school, whole family and whole world approach. We are always looking at unifying and bringing together, working in unity with those around us and the world around us. When the soul is integrated in its society, with the mind and the body, then we come into a harmonious state, *santosha* (contentment, the second *niyama*).[4]

For professionals working with young people, this holistic approach ticks all the boxes: spiritual, physical, mental and social wellness – which have even been advocated by Ofsted (Office for Standards in Education, Children's Services and Skills),[5] and incidentally also fit neatly into the PSHE (personal, social, health,

3 Gambhirananda 2010.

4 The *yamas* and the *niyamas* are the social ethical codes and the personal moral codes in yoga, which we will explain later in the book.

5 Department for Education 2014.

economic education)[6] curriculum of self-care – because, as we know, yoga in its purest form (according to the eight limbs) addresses the whole person, going straight to the core of who we are, and heals us from the inside out rather than medicating the symptoms, which is the frustration of many a medic in the UK today as well as their poor patients.

Preconceptions

There are many preconceptions about yoga and we will meet them in secondary schools, among teens and their parents. Certainly, I come across many different understandings of yoga in my courses.

You have come to this book because yoga has played an important role in your life. You have experienced the power of a sustained yoga practice in transforming your life. You are reading this because you wish to share this with young people. Your own practice lies at the very heart of your capacity to transform the lives of others. Maybe you practise predominantly asana, maybe some mindfulness or breathing techniques or maybe you find inspiration in the philosophy or in service of others and now you wish to integrate other aspects of yoga. Here I intend to outline how to do that in an informative, useful and effective way.

Intentions

The outcome of any attempt is deeply connected to the intention. So, at the beginning of every course, I ask the group to set an intention for their time together. Here are some examples:

> 'Supporting teens in discovering a safe space, drawing out their authentic, empowered selves to co-create a compassionate community.'
>
> 'To create a safe place in which teens can breathe and just be and give them lots of tools to access lifelong capacity for self-soothing.'
>
> 'Healing young people through yoga.'

---

6 PSHE is a planned but not defined programme to help young people develop fully as individuals and as members of families and social and economic communities.

'Sharing a wellbeing toolbox to live an optimal life.'

'Sharing a toolbox for life with teens.'

'Engage, embrace, empower.'

Even though each group comes from different backgrounds and different countries, the intention they set for the course and their work with teens is often very similar, that of, quite simply, sharing the toolbox of yoga with them for their own joy and optimal wellbeing.

At this stage it would be beneficial for you to set your own intention in reading the book and also in your work with teens, so that you are clear what you want from it. This way the book will be optimally beneficial to you. So, sit quietly for a minute or so and tune in with your deepest wish for young people and, when something has risen out of your heart, write it down in your journal.

Stepping into the breach

Every course I run attracts at least one medic and a few psychologists who are curious to start sharing yoga for young people. I believe that this is due to the rise in an acute awareness that we need to support young people to be optimally well so that we lessen the burden on the NHS and bring down the rate of lifestyle diseases from the current rate of 70 per cent![7]

There are also school teachers and teacher assistants on every course I run, and this is because, in the main, schools are now having to deal with quite severe cases of mental health difficulties, which in the past would have been quickly referred to CAMHS, such as schizophrenia and bipolar disorder. This is because CAMHS, in many instances, has seen up to 30 per cent cuts in the last few years so the waiting lists are long,[8] and the schools are expected to take care of the teens while they wait. The NHS is under tremendous pressure at a time when pharmaceutical companies are reaching ever younger children with drugs for depression, sleep problems and anxiety.[9]

7 Hughes 2016.
8 Forster 2017.
9 Torjesen 2016.

The rise in research in the field of yoga and also the interest and funding in mindfulness initiatives has prepared the ground for the work which you intend to undertake.

Your practice and your teaching

When Dr Cartwright of Westminster University started to look at the data extracted from the Big Yoga Survey which reached over 2000 practitioners through the UK, one thing jumped out at her – over 80 per cent of the respondents said that yoga had changed their lives in some major way – that is, they had either given up meat, alcohol, drugs or cigarettes or all four, or taken up other kinds of exercise.[10] They started making changes to their lifestyle which would ensure less suffering in the future and a higher likelihood of a healthy old age. General practitioners (GPs) often bemoan the fact that they request their patients to change their lifestyle in order to ensure a healthy life, but only a very small percentage, under 20 per cent, actually manage to make any changes at all. How did yoga change your life? You have chosen to become a teacher, I wonder what propelled you to take that choice?

Most students who come on my course do so because they love yoga so much, they have a hunger to go deeper, find out more and ensconce themselves in the practice on a regular basis. Very few of them actually come for purely practical or professional reasons! I hope your teacher training course gave you a chance to properly embed your yoga practice in your life; if it did, then I hope you also started to see your place in the world differently and relate to the people and the planet in a more compassionate and inclusive way.

Yoga is embodied literacy, it is being able to understand oneself, the world and others through the subtle listening of the body in various techniques. It is about becoming so in tune with our bodies that we can sense and work with issues before they have become tangible illnesses or handicaps in our daily life. We are literate about our bodies, we understand how our mind expresses itself through the body. We experience ourselves honestly and subtly with an open focus and without judgement. We are then able to integrate pain and joy, shadows and light, into an inclusive

10 Cartwright 2017.

and accepting individual who belongs to a healthy and vital community. When we are in tune to this degree we no longer make bad choices but instead choose optimal situations that serve us and the greater good.

A teacher needs to make sure their practice of yoga is fulfilling, correct and complete. Then their teaching will be effortless. I remember my Ayurvedic doctor coming to speak at a conference in 2016; he was the picture of wellness: calm, serene and complete. When asked if he had a PowerPoint to deliver he simply looked at me and said, 'I don't know what I am going to speak about yet.' On the day, he took some time on stage before speaking; he stood with everyone's eyes on him, fully focused, and simply told us a story about his evening. It was arguably the best lecture of the conference. In my opinion, he didn't actually need to say anything to teach us everything about Ayurveda. With this in mind, how do you embody yoga in your life?

When you are practising the full majesty of yoga, you will be aligned to your true purpose, to those around you and to the service of those who need you.

Summary

So, in summary, how can we be of service to young people who are struggling? The deeper you dive in yoga and in yourself, the more you have to offer, simple as that. When we are ignorant of our own ego and the desires that drive us forward at the expense of others then we cannot really make a positive difference.

I urge you to take a look at the *yamas* and the *niyamas*, the moral and ethical code of yoga. Not only is it a fabulous opportunity for reflection but it is also a great and interesting topic for conversation with young people! We will be touching on it in the second part as an idea for lesson planning.

Yoga is a complete practice, delving into ethical codes of conduct as well as social codes and internal value systems. It helps us use our breath in an intelligent way as well as to keep our bodies healthy. This complete approach needs to be the one we share, because, if we simply focus on the body, we are perpetuating a one-sided, materialist perspective on life, which is disturbing and destructive to so many young people.

Then you will be available to offer a richer understanding of yoga to the students and help them along the way with more tools. Most young people are at a crossroads, looking for meaning that makes sense of a changing world. The belief system of yoga is often separate from that of their parents and yet recognisable and non-threatening, as it is totally inclusive of all other religions and cultures; it certainly reflects and responds to the issues that they are experiencing. So, the philosophy of yoga might be a tool to help support the teens further. Yoga in its broadest sense is a new way of seeing the world which is fundamentally transformative.

The *yamas* and *niyamas* support their ability to choose correct behaviour and response to situations that arise. They support common sense and promote a fundamentally sensible way of life. In an increasingly secular society it is wonderful if these guidelines are introduced in some way, even if it is implicit, simply in your own behaviour. A society with healthy, positive and responsible young people is a society ready to take on the world; a society that questions the status quo and demands change lies at the heart of true democracy.

I hope to broaden your view on yoga, providing alternatives and options on how a yoga class for teens may look. Clearly, you need to be respectful of the situation you are in and what has been asked of you (school, youth centre), but there may be times when an asana practice could be substituted with a chanting session in some form, or a discussion on values and meaning. Can you imagine sharing yoga in another way, other than asana?

Yoga for teenagers is delightfully joyful and pleasurable with an underlying importance which cannot be overstated. I often asked myself the question to begin with, whether yoga was any different from gym, dance and rugby in its application to young people? I went deeply into the question: What do these young people get out of yoga which they don't get out of other sports? Is yoga simply a sport?

What do you think?

I want this book to take you gently out of your comfort zone, challenge your perceptions of yoga and also of young people, so that you can become a better teacher and maybe a more embodied yogi. I hope you will allow yourself to go on this adventure with me and explore the beauty and majesty of true yoga.

Thoughts to consider:

- How does yoga fit into your life?
- What do you mean by yoga?
- What do you think young people understand by yoga?
- What does the school or environment, where you intend to share yoga, understand by the term?
- What makes yoga different from any other sport or practice?

— Chapter 2 —

WHO ARE TEENS TODAY?

She cycles into school, unaware of her surroundings and in her own world of the dramas of school and social media. Suddenly, she becomes aware of someone whistling; looking around, she notices four men, hanging off the scaffolding on a building site, gawping, scanning her body, whistling and shouting at her. Flushed, nervous, it was the moment she realised that others saw her as a woman. No longer a child, she had been unceremoniously and innocently dragged into the world of sex and sexualisation. From then on, her relationship with her own body, men and boys in her class changed.

Identity – who are we in relation to the world?

The benefit of working with young people is that we have all been there. What do you remember? Do you remember shyness, infatuation, desire for excitement and closeness? Are you aware of the shift that happened for you from childhood to adulthood? The transition from innocence to self-awareness? Can you recall the pain of feeling alienated at a party where you didn't know anyone or becoming ostracised for wearing the 'wrong' clothes or liking the wrong music? How was it for you?

Please journal your responses before you carry on.

In this chapter we will get an idea of how the sands are shifting for young people. We will also discover some of the potential reasons for why we are experiencing a mental health crisis and how yoga might help to alleviate this and guide young people on a path of peace, both inward and outward.

Adolescent years have always been a challenging time, from Hamlet's anguish over his mother's sexuality to the passion and anger of today's young rock artists. Please reflect over which perennial issues have hounded young people through the generations. What makes them different from children? Why do so many school systems the world over move children at the age of 11 or 13 to a different school? In the past you transitioned from a child to an adult as soon as you had hair on your face or menstruated. What has changed? What are the differences between today's adolescents and yesterday's young adults?

Please take the opportunity to journal these answers.

The main psychological themes of these years for many are:

- fear of alienation/desire to belong
- rumination/anxiety
- concern with appearances
- desire to connect with others
- risky behaviour
- vitality
- rise in intellectual capacity
- separation from parents, desire for independence
- forming intimate bonds
- sex, sexuality, finding a partner
- being constantly switched on (online social media).

How are these different from your concerns as a teen?

What most of us don't understand is that these changes are biologically driven, socially enhanced and underlined by the biological imperative of looming adulthood. Becoming an adult, for some, is a painful procedure that comes way too soon and, for others, cannot come quickly enough! For some the moment of adolescence is a charmed independence where there is still support when needed.

Have you ever visited a cousin or a nephew once when they are around 11 and then when they turn 13 – what happened in the interim? What are these changes? Kevin in the 1990s UK TV sketch show *Harry Enfield and Chums*, who on his 13th birthday changes from an enthusiastic bouncing tigger to a monosyllabic monster in front of the doting eyes of his parents, is, for many of us, a very recognisable and puzzling shift. Many parents mourn the loss of the hugging, thoughtful, funny young girl or boy and are perplexed at this new strange being in their midst.

A time of change

The combination of chemical changes and societal expectations push the adolescent out of the house to find other groups to belong to; a bit like the cub in a lion pack, they start to roam free. When we perceive young people in the light of zoological phenomena, it is easier to understand the fundamental drivers of their behaviour and actions. It might also be easier to understand how much of what we do is conditioned by chemicals in our body. Anyone who has felt the urge to have a baby or fallen in love will know how that feels.

The hormonal changes herald the burgeoning unrecognisable physical body. From the adolescent perspective, it can feel a bit like this: I now bump my hips and shoulders in areas where before I slipped through with ease. I take up as much space as an adult and am treated accordingly. The invisible inner workings might not yet have caught up with my exterior, and this disconnect forms part of the anguish of a young person. Where there might still be a yearning for the comfort and support of the parents or carers, the physical body speaks of a different relationship. Where I might be sexualised by those around me, internally perhaps no such feelings are arising. Into this mix we add the intense desire to belong and fit in to whatever current social norm. As we leave our parents and make our way to parties and events by ourselves, it is essential for our survival that we belong to something else – that we have an alternative abode we can call home. Maybe that home is someone else's house, or maybe it's a club or a sport or an interest group. The desire to belong to this second group is so strong that we may well act in foolish ways to ensure our belonging. Remember the characters in the film *Grease*? Danny was a very different character with Sandy than he was with his mates – the vulnerability of the characters is often visible to the onlooker but not to the character. Alienation, for many, equals social death. See Albert Camus's *Outsider*,[1] a commonly read book for English exams for that very reason, as it explores the quality of being an outsider, someone who does not belong anywhere.

As our intellectual capacity rises during puberty, this means that we might be able to think more abstractly, theorise, understand complicated philosophical reasoning and consider others' feelings and situations better than before. However, the mind may not be in its optimal state because of lack of circadian rhythm (our inner 24-hour clock which differentiates between day and night), lack of sleep, lack of optimal nutrition, lack of a strong attachment figure or lack of guidance. Sleep is often the first thing to be disturbed during teen years, due to changes in melatonin, the sleep neurotransmitter, which regulates our sleep pattern, and also due to bedtime screen time. If we do not sleep enough (nine hours between 14 and 19 years old) there will be mood disturbances and mental health consequences. We also often start to cook and feed ourselves in different contexts, which can lead to suboptimal nutrition. If we have been brought up in a family with disturbing patterns of depression, alcoholism or absenteeism, then we might find it hard to form strong and lasting bonds with those around us, which in turn leads to difficulty in focusing and general intellectual performance (attachment theory).[2] Many parents, carers and friends are not sure how to support their teens at this age and may step back completely, leaving the youngster to fend for themselves, unguided and unclear of their path.

In these cases, there is often a rise in rumination and subsequent anxiety. From an Ayurvedic perspective, anxiety is often connected to lack of groundedness[3] and lack of connection with others.

> *Ayurveda* means the science of life and incorporates yoga, with many aspects of wellbeing including nutrition, movement, cleansing techniques, massages and various other ancient wellness sciences.

---

1 Camus 1942.

2 Attachment theory is John Bowlby's (1969) suggestion that babies come into the world biologically pre-programmed to form attachments with others as this helps them to survive.

3 Being grounded is a term often used in yoga and Ayurveda, meaning to feel connected to the earth and the body.

Grounded and connected

According to Ayurveda, anxiety can have many reasons, such as lack of being grounded – this can mean literally not spending enough time on the ground in nature, barefoot preferably, or it could mean not spending enough time in awareness of the body, whether in yoga asana, massage or similar techniques. It is often also the reason why we eat, to feel our bodies and our connection to it – especially if we spend a lot of time in our heads, with the mental work that school demands.

The connection with others is something that is a need in every living being and determines whether we thrive or not. Interconnectedness is an integral part of yoga, as we said earlier, bringing all aspects together, whether it be our mind with our body, or our neighbourhood or countries. Feeling connected to each other lies at the heart of wellness. I often translate yoga to the word connection. For example, recent fascinating research proves that women who had many friends had a lower risk of Type 2 diabetes than those who felt lonely.[4]

Online and disconnected

Emerging studies are showing an alarming relationship between increased (online) connectivity and anxiety in young people.[5] I watch the young people I work with – constantly checking the phone, never completely present – as their awareness is always being drawn outwards away from their present experience by each vibration or ping. In Buddhism, as in yoga and mindfulness, joy is to be found in the present moment. When our mind is constantly being drawn outwards, it is fractured, caught up in others' opinions, feelings and attitudes, attached to both pain and pleasure, riding the rollercoaster of emotions. Our fear of being judged and desire to belong are constantly being fired up, with every waking moment filled with tension and an outward-looking perspective.

Obviously, the upside of connectivity could be that we have our friends only a click away – we can actually see them in real

---

4 Brinkhues *et al.* 2017.

5 Turkle 2012.

time as they cook, sleep or work. This sense of never being alone is comforting at best and fulfils the teen's desire to belong.

However, there have been too many situations of cyber-bullying with my students to ignore the matter here. The moment when your friends post a video of you being beaten up, shamed or ridiculed is a moment which for some has led to suicide. The addiction to the online presence is something which is changing our lives on so many levels; the level of trust among young people is changing, the meaning of intimacy, the meaning of friendship and the meaning of trust.

This dangerous cocktail of the desire to connect and to belong together, with the fear of alienation, married to the inherent risky behaviour pattern, can bring about disastrous choices. Naked shots being sent to the boy I fancy, who then posts them for everyone to see, sexting at an early age, the porn readily available on any smartphone – all of which plays havoc with our burgeoning sexuality.

Summary

When we understand that adolescents first need to belong to a group, second, need to connect with others and, third, need to take risks, then maybe we can harness these fundamental drives and gather them in a different direction that is more engaging, edifying, fascinating and beneficial in the long term. When we can truly meet those needs with integrity, through exciting and fun yoga classes which challenge and take risks, within their abilities, eventually drawing them inwards towards introspection, then I believe that these online experiences will drop away, no longer central to their lives, as has happened to many of my students.

> *When I do yoga, I'm so caught up in the moment that I forget to look at my phone, my friends get angry with me 'cos I never turn it on.* (Edie, 18)[6]

On many of my courses, therapists and psychiatrists echo the same fear, namely that young people cannot abide the thought or

---

6 Bainbridge 2017.

the fact of being alone. This fear of being with oneself must have repercussions. If we are not comfortable in our own skin, with our minds, delving deep into our own soul, then what hope have we of feeling fulfilled or content?

It seems to me that the optimal response to this frantic outward-looking phenomenon would be to introduce introspection. Can we guide young people in a physical practice towards patience and stillness within themselves until they feel safe enough to be still in their own soul? This practice is what I call yoga.

When we move away from constant distraction and come into the place of stillness, many of us discover our true passion, our true voice, and are able to relate to others from a unique place, without the need to lose ourselves in the group. Rooted in stillness we are able to co-regulate effectively, effortlessly bringing peace to others as well as ourselves. Then we come to the realisation of our own value or meaning in our life. We receive the silent responses to questions such as: What do I have to give? How much more am I than my physical appearance?

Then ensues a lifetime journey towards optimal wellbeing, full acceptance of what is and complete acceptance of others as well as ourselves.

— Chapter 3 —

WHAT GOES ON IN THE BRAIN OF A TEEN?

> It was the day before her exam. Mike had just passed his test and got a new Yamaha bike. He texted her, 'Let's go for a ride along the river, I'll pick you up in quarter of an hour!' Mike was handsome and popular, and she really liked him. Without hesitation she said yes. She sneaked out, her mum shouting, 'Where are you going? It's late and you've got your exam in the morning.' Ignoring the calls, she rushed out into the darkness and jumped on the back of the big blue machine waiting outside and sped off. The sound of the powerful engine, her arms around his waist, she had never felt so free! The exam could wait, she'd do an all-nighter!

Only a few years before, Linda would not have considered acting so impetuously, nor would she just a few years later. But with the brain in its adolescent phase, she was up for taking risks, dropping revision and feeling independent. These actions are neurologically encoded.

The neuroscience of adolescence

Have you ever wondered what causes the abrupt and mostly unwelcome metamorphosis of your child in the teenage years? Acting impetuously, contrary to common sense? Why have they become extra secretive or why do they see you as the enemy when before you were their closest ally? Have they become curious about drugs, sex, the meaning of life? Take a moment to reflect in your journal about the cognitive (brain) changes you have noticed in your teen or those that you know. Wouldn't you like to know what is happening in the brain?

In this book we are taking a holistic look at the development during adolescence and taking together the different aspects of development. The brain is the locus of substantial change – in this chapter we will explore the numerous changes that take place there.

Nature or nurture – is this person the product of her environment, friends and family or is she simply hardwired to behave in this way because of her chemical make-up? It is a combination of the two. The mind is the whole organism that is being used to respond to an event; the mind resides in the body, the whole body helps us make a decision – not just the brain, which in fact has only a small impact.

'My mind is made up; my mind is unclear; to my mind, she is at fault.' What do we mean by the word 'mind'? Some of us immediately equate mind with brain but the mind is far more than that. How do we make up our minds? What are the factors that play into mood, mind and brain? What is the connection between mind and body?

The chemical constellation of our brain, our mind and our bodies is intrinsic to the way we behave. When we are lacking in a particular chemical or mineral our entire personality can change. For example, have you ever experienced anaemia (lack of iron) – you become lethargic, sleepy, fuzzy headed? Or if you have ever known anyone who lacks B6 or B12, they can become anxious or depressed? Omega 3, 6 and 9 help us think clearly and quickly. The list goes on. Not only does what we eat or not eat affect our body, but also our mind.

The mind is made up of various chemical impulses from all over the body, mostly the gut and the brain, but also various important nerves that activate and enervate various parts, for example the vagus nerve, which travels from point to point in the body and is both afferent and efferent, meaning it is sending messages both up and down all the time, bringing in information from all parts of the body and sending messages to the brain and vice versa.

Whereas the intellect is finite and limited by experience and knowledge, insight and intuition are part of a deeper and more mysterious wisdom, which indicates a connection to something far deeper, more majestic and far more imaginative than the limited intellect. This wisdom and insight can be a lifeline for many young people who feel lost and exceedingly influenced by others and the outside world. We need to take a look at what is happening in the brain and mind to fully understand the massive shifts and changes taking place at this time.

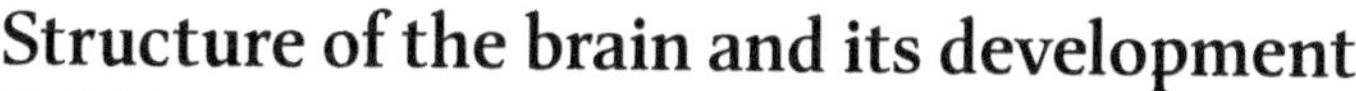

Structure of the brain and its development

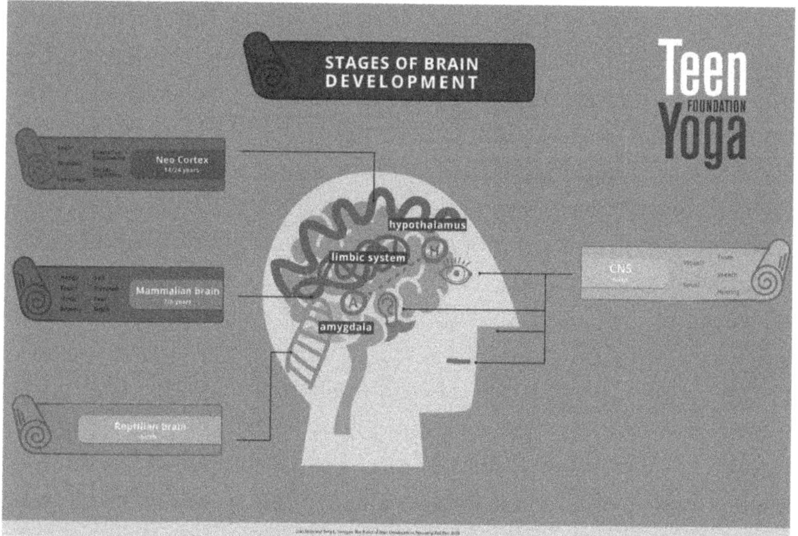

Imagine for a moment the development of a foetus from a single cell, or the development of a baby into a toddler, the amount of skills that are learned and how many changes take place in order for those skills to be accomplished. There are three major stages of development in a human being's lifetime: foetus, toddlerhood and adolescence.

What happens in this time? In utero, the foetus develops from a single cell to a human being in nine months – a cell grows organs, limbs, brain and nervous system, enough to survive in the outside world! Toddlers move from helpless beings into someone who can function in the world by themselves. Babies are helpless, they need feeding, nappies changing, even putting to sleep. As a toddler, we can do all these things by ourselves, we have learnt how to walk, talk, poo and eat by ourselves in a relatively short period of time. Imagine the amount of brain power needed to achieve these goals and make these changes! What is extraordinary is that similar amounts of neurons (nerve cells) are being deposited in the brain and across the entire nervous system during adolescence. At only three times in our lives do this many neurons become available for us to use, in utero, in toddlerhood and adolescence. So what does this mean?

Not only do we have an abundance of neurons available for our use in the teenage years (how we use them is another matter) but we are also learning how to function from a more reasoned and reflective state of mind, so the brain is not only in neurogenesis (making new structures) but it is also neuroplastic – it is changing what is there and utilising different parts in new ways that are adapted to the outside world. These changes are completely dependent on nurture. What are we experiencing at this time? What are we learning? We have an enormous capacity for learning and it is used in order to position ourselves in relation to society and the world around us. As a foetus, the neurons are used to create a physical body and mind. As a toddler, they are used to create a functioning human. As an adolescent, they are used to create a functioning human in society.

The nervous system is already developing in the first three weeks of foetal life, at a very rapid rate. Nerve cells multiply and migrate to take their place in the system, guided by a scaffold of supportive glial cells. By the end of the second trimester of pregnancy this process is largely complete, with clear patterns of structural organisation and functional differentiation visible. Development continues more slowly throughout life in the womb, and afterwards; the nervous system is not fully mature until at least 20 years after birth.

There is a very clear choreography and precise order to this development. For instance, the myelin sheaths necessary for rapid information transmission begin to develop around the nerves in the limbs, and myelination gradually proceeds along the spinal cord towards the brain stem, with the visual nerves becoming myelinated in the first few months after birth, and the nerves controlling movement becoming fully myelinated around 18 months of age. (Myelination is when a nerve becomes covered with fatty tissue to make it more effective.) In the cerebral cortex myelination progresses from the back of the brain to the front of the brain.[1]

1 The cerebral cortex is the largest part of the cerebrum in the brain; it is the outer layer of grey matter and is found only in mammals. It is generally classified into four lobes: frontal, parietal, temporal and occipital lobes.

After birth the brain continues to grow, more than doubling in weight during the baby's first year of life. The brain continues to grow more slowly until around 12–15 years of age, and myelination also continues. The organisation of the nerve cells in the brain grows in complexity throughout childhood and adolescence: at birth each nerve cell has 7500 connections and these increase rapidly until there are double the connections in an adult brain, but weak connections are then 'pruned' away.

We used to think that brain circuits were inalterable once development was complete, but it is now known that the brain continues to reallocate circuits and synapses[2] throughout life (neuroplasticity), although it will never again be as flexible as during childhood and adolescence. In the first six years of life, a child develops new skills more rapidly than they ever will again, as the nervous system organises itself to enable movement, language and growing autonomy. This process then slows down until, during adolescence, there is another surge in development as new sophisticated skills of social awareness and judgement emerge.

The internally directed process of neurological development is modified by experience and life circumstances. The basic structure of the nervous system is elaborated according to experience and learning to create and strengthen neural synapses and circuits. We call this process *neuroplasticity*, and it follows a rule of 'use it or lose it' or, more positively, 'use it and grow it'. Brain circuits are increasingly allocated to any interest that we focus on persistently – for instance, researchers have tracked the changes in the brains of London taxi drivers studying for 'the knowledge' test in order to become black cab drivers; brain circuits that are unused get reallocated to other functions.[3]

In the developing brain, the 'use it or lose it' rule is unforgiving, as the brain has only a limited time period to fine tune its major structural organisation, and major deficits will not be repairable; for example, a child who has not learned language by the end of the first critical period will never develop language skills fully.

There are three critical periods during development when synaptic formation and cerebral cortex maturation depends on

2 A synapse is a junction between two nerve cells, consisting of a minute gap across which electrical impulses pass.

3 Maguire, Woollett and Spiers 2006.

appropriate experience, and during which the plasticity of the brain is maximal. The first year of life is a critical period for maturation of the *sensorimotor* cortex. During the subsequent seven or eight years there is a critical period for the maturation of the *temporal*, *occipital* and *parietal* areas of the cerebral cortex, underpinning vision and hearing and the acquisition of language and musicality. The final critical period occurs during adolescence, and this final increase in neuroplasticity enables the maturation of the *prefrontal cortex*.

The prefrontal cortex

This area of the cerebral cortex is responsible for the most complex cognitive skills. The trend throughout neurodevelopment is for more complex skills, and their underlying neural circuits, to mature later; areas that process more complex information are 'trained' by experiences which only become possible later once simpler skills are mastered. Similarly, earlier in life we see that areas of the cerebral cortex responsible for processing sound mature earlier than the language areas.

The prefrontal cortex matures in the context of a social group and an environment that enables experimentation with making decisions and judgements, and with taking risks. These experiences are necessary to enable the development of mature executive function. Earlier in life there has been no need to exercise these skills if competent parents have been available to perform these functions. Where parents are not able to adequately fulfil these functions, and young people have to attempt to take on responsibilities before the prefrontal cortex matures, it places them under stress.

The prefrontal cortex is responsible for planning, organising and regulating complex activity, with areas specialised for maintaining attention, self-control and impulse inhibition and emotional decision-making. It is vitally important in social judgement, communication, abstract thinking, risk assessment and decision-making, and expression of personality. Working memory (the ability to hold information in mind and manipulate it, for instance during mental arithmetic) is also dependent on the prefrontal cortex.

The skills that rely on the prefrontal cortex are often referred to generally as *executive function*, due to their importance in differentiating between conflicting options, making sense of moral and ethical conundrums, imagining possible outcomes of actions and planning activities that support future goals.

The prefrontal cortex also enables vital social skills such as understanding other people's experience and point of view, awareness of emotional expression, understanding of social rules about inappropriate behaviour and ability to monitor and control one's own social behaviour.

Neurodevelopment during adolescence

Increased neuroplasticity during adolescence reflects the further organisation of nerve cell connections and circuits; increased myelination of nerve axons,[4] further pruning of synapses and changes in neurotransmitter systems occur during this final critical period of neurodevelopment. The changes in the levels of sex hormones at the onset of puberty play an important role in triggering and coordinating this process.

While connections between brain areas become stronger (resulting in growth in white matter), pruning of excess nerve cells (improving efficiency at the expense of some flexibility) results in the grey matter shrinking slightly; measurement of the thickness of the cerebral cortical grey matter has found that it peaks during adolescence before thinning to adult levels.

As this final critical period of development largely focuses on the prefrontal cortex, one might expect adolescence to be characterised by a steady improvement in executive functions, but this is not what we observe. There can instead appear to be a reduction in executive function in comparison to earlier stages of neurodevelopment, which can be frustrating for parents and adolescents. However, this makes logical sense when we realise that the prefrontal cortex is largely functional prior to the final neurodevelopmental surge in adolescence; the changes during this period are to a large extent 'fine tuning' of existing skills, with a consequent apparent loss of skills as connections are loosened. Therefore, the changes in the brain during this period of development result in a pattern of

4 A nerve axon is a long thread-like part of a nerve cell along which impulses are conducted from the cell body to other cells.

less focused brain activity than is seen in the adult brain during problem solving. This is necessary for enabling the flexibility to create new neural circuits (for example, learning how to select the 'best' behaviour according to the situation) but results in less efficient thinking patterns until the 'best' circuits are selected for survival during the pruning process.

This relative inefficiency means that the 'executive load' tends to increase in adolescents; they may not be consciously aware that their brains are not working as well as they used to, but they are often aware that everything seems like harder work than it used to. This means that adolescents can be at risk of *chronic stress*, which has its own negative effects on brain function.

While this account might suggest that adolescents lose previously learned skills, this is not the case. In some circumstances, particularly when the perceived benefits are high, adolescents can demonstrate mature planning and self-organisation skills. There is however an imbalance between the maturation of these skills, which have been described as 'cold' cognition, and the emotional decision-making functions, or 'hot' cognition, which is thought to be involved in adolescents' relatively poor risk assessment and decision-making skills in emotional or social contexts.

Emotional decision-making appears to mature later than other executive abilities, although some researchers have argued that the two systems usually work together but can compete when adolescents are emotionally highly aroused.[5] Researchers have demonstrated that adolescents apply their risk assessment skills more effectively and maturely when alone than when in a group of their peers, for instance; this is not seen in adults or younger children.[6]

These changes in the adolescent brain are not occurring in isolation. At the same time most adolescents are facing increased pressure in school, in social groups and in their own self-organisation. They are often taking on new interests and new roles; some of these they have a choice about and some they don't. Puberty is an additional stress, as they have to navigate the physical changes it brings, as well as the dysregulation in their arousal levels,

5 Reyna and Farley 2006.

6 Knoll *et al.* 2015.

daily rhythms and sleep cycle that can result in a general feeling of imbalance.

Recently puberty has also been shown to be implicated in changes in the facial recognition system, which undergoes a retuning process to identify and gravitate towards people at a similar stage of puberty; before puberty children's facial recognition systems are orientated towards adult women, or mother figures. This is occurring at a time when ability to identify expressed emotion is still developing.

Some people have argued that these changes and stresses play a vital role in enabling adolescents to learn effective and mature self-regulatory skills. In earlier life, competent parents would have helped manage the demands of school and social life, supporting organisation and acting to an extent as a surrogate prefrontal cortex. From this perspective, the greater activation of the emotional brain in adolescence, with a greater response to anticipated reward and a reduced sensitivity to punishment, would support the adolescent in their movement towards autonomy and away from safety. This would parallel the importance of curiosity in early childhood when it enables toddlers to overcome their fear and explore their environment.

Although autonomy is the goal of this period of development, it is better thought of as *interdependence* rather than independence; humans are social in nature, and brain organisation reflects this with large areas of cortex devoted to emotional and social processes. The developing links between the prefrontal cortex and the *limbic system* are heavily influenced by the adolescent's interaction with their parents, reflecting the importance of maintaining family relationships during this period.[7]

The effects of stress and trauma

Adolescence is a very stressful period, and a lot of young people find it difficult to cope, particularly if they have experienced trauma. Abuse, stress and trauma all stimulate the body's emergency systems, acutely and chronically, and impact negatively on neurodevelopment.

---

7 Also known as the mammalian brain, the limbic system is the centre of several important structures in the brain that all work together to regulate some of the brain's most important processes.

We can think of stress as just being under too much pressure – trying to carry too much – and becoming gradually exhausted as a result. In the end, everything becomes a challenge and a potential emergency.

How does the body and brain respond to stress?

The body's monitoring system has a very effective red alert system. An emergency, particularly a threat to the self, immediately activates the *sympathetic nervous system* and triggers the release of the hormone adrenaline from the adrenal glands into the blood system.[8] Just like when the red alert siren goes off in a film, on a warship or spaceship of some kind, adrenaline diverts all the body's resources to defence and attack, abandoning the day-to-day tasks and routine maintenance.

Chronic stress is more like an ongoing 'yellow alert' – like a warship on patrol, constantly on the alert, unable to stand down. After months on 'yellow alert', working double shifts with short rations, the warship crew will be exhausted and bad tempered, and the ship itself may have issues, as no one has had time for routine maintenance tasks. Similarly, chronic stress takes its toll on the body as there is no downtime for maintenance and repair; the adrenaline system works well for managing acute emergencies but the body does not function well in continuous emergency mode.

Unfortunately, we often perpetuate a 'yellow alert' state by thinking about our problems, as the limbic system is old, in evolutionary terms, and cannot tell the difference between a real threat and an imaginary threat; film makers exploit this in thrillers and horror films – if it weren't for this 'glitch', watching *Psycho* would be as enthralling as watching paint dry.

The main hormone underlying the chronic stress response is cortisol, which is also released from the adrenal glands. It is a hormone that is intricately involved in the control of metabolism (the extraction of energy from food) and is vital for life. Cortisol is released throughout the day. Cortisol levels are lowest during the

8 The sympathetic nervous system is one of the two main divisions of the autonomic nervous system, the other being the parasympathetic nervous system. These regulate the body's unconscious actions. The sympathetic nervous system's primary process is to stimulate the body's fight or flight reaction.

night and highest early in the morning, making it easier for us to wake up. When there is persisting stress or an ongoing emergency, cortisol levels increase and the pattern of release changes so that levels remain high throughout the day. This increases the amount of glucose in the blood, reduces the immune response and can have a toxic effect on nerve cells, particularly those involved in memory and long-term learning.

In addition to the exhaustion, fatigue and general malaise caused by chronic stress, there are specific effects on the nervous system. Psychologically, stress and anxiety can also inhibit experimentation and learning, which may result in the prefrontal cortex not developing fully before the end of the critical period of neuroplasticity.

The persistently high levels of cortisol interfere with the function of the hypothalamic-pituitary-adrenal axis (HPA axis)[9] and the autonomic nervous system (see Chapter 6), which can impact on homeostasis (the inherent balance in the body).

Adolescents can appear to lose prior skills; however, this is temporary during the acquisition of new skills of emotional decision-making, social judgement and abstract thought. This process is stressful and arduous and requires active involvement by the adolescent, triggered by increased levels of motivation and novelty seeking (without which it would be tempting not to bother). Significant difficulties during this period occur with making decisions under emotional or social stress.

Although many of these new skills relate to finding their place in the wider social and occupational world, development of the emotional brain proceeds more rapidly when communication with parents remains open.

The changes we observe during adolescence represent the outer manifestations of the final critical period of neurological development, during which substantial fine tuning of sophisticated and vital neural circuits occurs.

---

9 The HPA axis is in charge of the stress response in the body and 'switches on' the sympathetic nervous system throughout the body, releasing cortisol in the adrenals.

The teen brain and society

So, as we see, our brains and minds develop in tandem and are interacting with our social development. If we find ourselves in a 'safe' and inspiring environment, our brain is likely to develop more quickly and more effectively than if the inspiration or safety were lacking.

As we look for autonomy and independence first, creating a clear identity which can have something to offer society, so that we can then engage in a satisfying interdependence, we are equally dependent on our parents as we were during toddlerhood in terms of practising the use of our prefrontal cortex. Parents take the place of our prefrontal cortex until we have one ourselves! Independence is never a true goal of any mammal, but rather the interdependence on and trust of others of the same species to work together, collaborate and feel compassion. These values underpin a yoga practice, as we look to create a radical self-care programme for young people in order that they may be fully present in society. When we are able to collaborate in a satisfactory and egalitarian way, we move towards common goals, which are socially stated. We then become a fully fledged part of the future society we are in the process of building. We are trusted by and trusting of the people around us, to deliver and adapt to each other.

A functioning society is one where we work as one, just as the cells of a body work together to create a functioning organism. As John Donne says:

> No man is an island, entire of itself; every man is a piece of the continent, a part of the main. If a clod be washed away by the sea, Europe is the less, as well as if a promontory were, as well as if a manor of thy friend's or of thine own were: any man's death diminishes me, because I am involved in mankind, and therefore never send to know for whom the bell tolls; it tolls for thee.[10]

Psychologically, this can only happen when we feel safe. Psychological safety means we trust the people around us to deliver and support us in times of difficulty, when we feel able to open up about doubts or fears to the people around us. If we have these kinds of secure attachments, we will build psychological resilience and do better in life (see the following graphic).

---

10 'No Man Is an Island', by John Donne, Meditation 17, from *Devotions upon Emergent Occasions*, 1624.

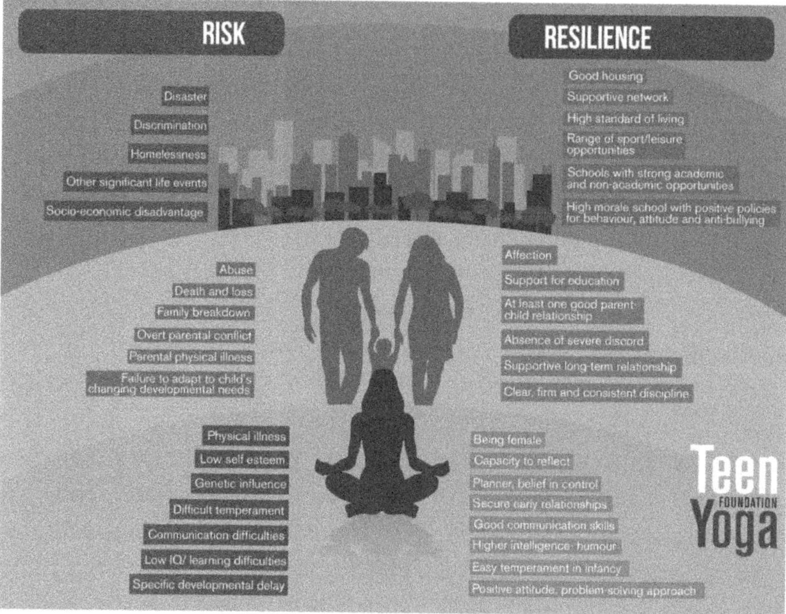

As you can see, resilience to stress is largely determined by social factors. So, in summary, there is a direct correlation between resilience and trust.

It is misconceived to believe that if anything 'bad' happens to me, then I will be more at risk. In fact, stressors are often what make us resilient. The 'right' amount of stress builds strength and resilience, whereas stress above and beyond what I can cope with will lead to a risk factor. We might be able to draw a parallel with nature, where a tree on a windy ledge will become stronger through the battle with the elements. However, if you transplant a weak sapling onto the top of a windy hill, it is likely to break and die.

So we can conclude that stress is a natural part of adolescence. The way the brain develops, coupled with the expectations of those around us in society and the expectations we have of ourselves, creates enough stress to ensure change and a certain amount of necessary resilience to move into adulthood. One could say that the mismatches between these two areas create a certain stress.

The million-dollar question is, how do we respond to stress? Do we have the capacity to relax and deal with the situation or do we crack under the slightest bit of pressure? The individual who can take life in their stride, at ease, moving slowly towards each challenge with confidence, will become stronger and more resilient, whereas the one who breaks under the first stressful event will be at risk for many problems further down the line.

How yoga impacts the brain in adolescence

What yoga does, in this very specific context, is take the first step towards wellbeing, which is to teach us how to respond intelligently and effectively to stressful situations by using the breath and adopting certain attitudes which programme us to positivity.

When cortisol is coursing through the body over a longer period of time (chronic stress), certain limitations occur in the brain – the size of the hippocampus (area of learning and memory) shrinks, the connections to the prefrontal cortex are not made, the size of the prefrontal cortex is smaller than it could be, the size of the brain is smaller in general and the connections between the right and left side of the brain are not made to such a large degree. This is because when we are under constant threat the development during adolescence is focused on the limbic area of the brain, which is the fear area. No time or space is given to development of memory or executive function.[11]

How many times have we had students, adult or young, who, after coming to yoga, say, 'I feel so relaxed – I sleep so well after yoga!'? This is because a yoga class has two main effects on the nervous system – it reduces the cortisol in the blood by down-regulating the sympathetic nervous system (we will go into more detail about this in Chapter 6) and it releases gamma-aminobutyric acid (GABA), which is the anti-anxiety neurotransmitter in the brain.[12]

Cortisol is the main culprit in stress; it is released into the blood so that we can flee or fight. It takes some other action for it to be released out of the body: deep breathing, gentle movement or meditation, otherwise it stays in the muscles and blood stream for up to 72 hours. When we are constantly under stress, the body never relaxes and allows itself to repair and restore. When we learn certain techniques, we can consciously manage the cortisol production, allowing the body to come into healing mode more quickly and efficiently, thereby protecting it from harm.

---

11 Robinson *et al.* 2013.

12 Gangadhar 2013; Streeter *et al.* 2010.

GABA, a powerful neurotransmitter in the brain, alleviates anxiety effectively and quickly. Chris Streeter's research on this is interesting and requires further study: 'The 12-week yoga intervention was associated with greater improvements in mood and anxiety than a metabolically matched walking exercise. This is the first study to demonstrate that increased thalamic GABA levels are associated with improved mood and decreased anxiety.'[13]

Also, there is a certain vagus nerve stimulation, in some backward-bending postures primarily, which stimulates the parasympathetic nervous system (see Porges's research on this).[14] According to Porges's theory, the vagus nerve is an important player in the effectiveness of asana and breathing practice in changing mood. The vagus nerve carries information back and forth from the brain and body, shifting mood states as part of its role, which is partly why psychiatrists still use vagal stimulation to support deeply depressed patients.[15]

In conclusion, stressed people benefit from yoga, both mentally and physically, through the reduction and conscious management of the stress response. The brain of the adolescent is very prone to stress responses for all the factors that we discussed earlier, so yoga at this age is particularly helpful. If we learn to cope with situations and control our responses to lower our stress reaction, we support a healthy brain growth and allow ourselves to adapt well to society and create a benevolent and compassionate outlook which will then form the basis of our future character, building a peaceful and understanding society for our future. As it is stated in the Chandogya Upanishad:

> You are what your deep driving desire is. As your desire is, so is your intention. As your intention is, so is your will. As your will is, so is your deed. As your deed is, so is your character. As your character is, so is your destiny.[16]

---

13 Streeter *et al.* 2010.

14 Porges 2001.

15 When I worked at the Callington Road Hospital in Bristol, service users would often come in having experienced a vagal stimulation by electric impulses to relieve depressive symptoms. This is a commonly used intervention in mental health in the UK today, as I understand it.

16 Krishnananda 2006.

— Chapter 4 —

THE CHANGING BODY

> When my son and I arrived at the cabin for our annual holiday – he was 14 years old – he ran into the loo and couldn't find the switch; he came back out – 'The light switch has moved!' he said. As he had grown almost 11 cm in a year, his hand reached too high on the wall. He had the impression that objects had shifted in space.

The key reason for this is proprioception. Our brain is constantly telling us where we are in relation to others and things around us. When we grow quickly, this proprioceptive ability doesn't quite catch up and we find ourselves bumping into things as we take up more room than we think.

Anatomical changes

In this chapter we will take a look at how the physical body changes and the impact this has on young people.

Adolescence is the time from puberty to adulthood. It can be roughly divided into three stages:

1. Early adolescence 11–13
2. Middle adolescence 14–16
3. Late adolescence 17–25

The body is constantly changing; it is a flow of rejuvenation, change and decay – our body morphs and changes to adapt to outer circumstances, in response to the needs and requirements of the outer and inner world. As with our mind, the body is a reflection of our habits, thoughts and attitudes. Adolescence is certainly a time when these attitudes and shapes are shaped for the rest of our lives. I remember when I worked as a school teacher, and parents would come in for parents' evening, I could often tell whose parent they were, because they would have the same mannerisms, stance or gait as their offspring! This is more than mimicry, this is an example of how we adopt the world view of our parents, expressed in our physical stance.

Can you remember how you felt about your body, growing up? Were you an early developer or a late one? I was late; I remember stuffing socks in my bra, to look more developed. I also remember asking for tampons, even though I didn't have my period yet, because being developed was desirable and exciting! I know that some of my friends were extremely embarrassed about developing too quickly; their breasts were in the way and heavy while taking part in sport, or having boys ogling them, when inside they still felt like children. This is an example of the awkward stage between physical maturation and inner development!

Young women, in general, develop more quickly than young men, giving rise to the awkward period between 11 and 15 of girls being taller and stronger than their male counterparts for a few years. In general women tend to have their growth spurt between 12 and 13, whereas boys have theirs between 14 and 15.

In the foetus the main body grows first, then the limbs grow. In adolescence it is the opposite way around, the feet and hands grow first, followed by the limbs. This is why, as parents and teachers, we notice big shoes before the person actually grows in height. It is an early indicator to buy longer trousers!

Growth and postural development

When we start to grow quickly and those around us stay the same it impacts on the way we stand, sit and move. What do you think might happen if you were the first to grow tall and you were taller than everyone else?

Can you tell a yogi, standing at a bus stop or sitting in a café? I notice that yogis tend to sit away from the backrest in chairs or release tension in their shoulders while waiting for a bus! These tendencies are a direct result of their daily or weekly asana practice.

We become more attuned to the needs for tension release and are constantly making little adjustments to address them.

The effects on our posture are telling – we tend to hunch to make ourselves smaller, to fit in and belong; as we have said – connection is the main driver. Whereas, if we are short, we tend to puff out our chest in an attempt to seem taller. These postural shifts also have an impact on our emotions and, in the long term, our character. Try it out for yourself – bring both shoulders forward, as if to protect your heart, bring your chin to your chest and notice how this makes you feel. Now do the opposite, puff out your chest, look up – notice how this makes you feel.

Bones grow and muscles grow and stretch – bones are a continuum of tissue from hard to soft. Babies' bones are relatively soft and malleable and, as we grow, they become harder (ossify). We know when someone has fully grown, as the phalanges in the fingers come together; this is a way to know whether someone has come to their full height or not.

As with the brain, how we spend our time determines how our bones grow and, in particular, the density of the bone as we grow. There will also be genetic and societal factors that play in to the growth, stature and height of an adolescent.

In girls the pelvis widens, while in young men the pectoral area and chest widen. In girls more fat deposits occur, while in young men fat becomes muscle.

If the pelvis widens quickly, it can lead to knock knees and flat feet among many girls. These postural anomalies can be corrected through yoga practices that help minimise the curve in the small of the back, turn the legs out and lift through the arch of the foot. If we leave these issues unaddressed, they can cause long-term damage and pain to the adult. However, if we develop a postural awareness at an early age, we can support a healthier and more conscious growth pattern that might support the alleviation of pain right from the start.

Can you think of any postures that might help a young woman whose pelvis has widened too quickly so that she is developing flat feet or knock knees?

Exercises to help with flat feet and knock knees

Flat feet: Curl the toes under as you kneel, to accentuate the arch; it might hurt at first, but be patient and do this exercise for a few minutes every day. It is the fascia at the base of the foot which is stretching.

Knock knees: Encourage outward rotation of hips, as well as flattening of spine against the floor. Wide-angle forward bend with conscious outward rotation and butterfly postures are good for this as well as moving bridge.

Posture

When we encounter someone who stands upright with their gaze at the horizon or naturally straight at you, we experience them as confident and respected. However, when we encounter someone with their head hidden, maybe in a hoodie, shoulders thrust forward and head down, avoiding our gaze, wanting to be invisible, remain unjudged, unseen, they can seem threatening.

When we start to practise asana, we are in fact practising attitudes as well as exercising our body and stretching certain areas. We practise how it might feel to open our chest or open our heart. We practise the attitude of gratitude as we open up. We practise the attitude of inward looking in the child posture, we practise balancing thoughts and emotions on a one-leg balance.

Our bodies are outer expressions of our inner world. With some practice, our postures bring us into harmony and balance; we exercise a balance of openings (curiosity and positivity) and nourishing 'closing' postures such as forward bends, we balance powerful arm balances with nurturing resting postures, and so on. In this way we balance all aspects of ourselves.

Back problems

On a more concrete note, you will come across young people with three main spinal issues: lordosis, kyphosis and scoliosis.

LORDOSIS

Lordosis is common among young gymnasts and ballerinas as well as in Afro Caribbean bodies. This is when the lower back has an exaggerated curve resulting in an open chest and the gaze naturally looking above the horizon. When this student is standing straight, sometimes the hands can end up hanging naturally behind the hips. How do you think we can help 'correct' this posture to avoid lower back pain or neck pain in the future?

For many Afro Caribbean women, this is not something to be corrected but is their correct posture.

- What would be the long-term issues with keeping this posture, both emotionally and physically?
- Have a think and make some notes on which postures might help with lordosis.
- You might like to think about which muscle groups are weak and which are strong in order for this posture to be present.

Some reasons why a teenager might have lordosis:

- muscle weakness in abdomen
- overcompensating muscles in the lower back
- dancing
- gymnastics
- attitude of pride or overcompensation
- short stature.

With this group you need to be sure you don't exaggerate backward bends and encourage straight, measure-forward bends and core engagement in all leg lifts and other postures.

Exercises to reduce lordosis

Pigeon is perfect for rounding the back a little and releasing pressure and tension in the buttocks and lower back.

KYPHOSIS

This posture is also known as hunchback and is when the upper back has an exaggerated curve, resulting in shoulders coming forward and a cave-like chest. The hands will end up hanging in front of the body in a natural position for those with kyphosis.

- Can you think of what might have caused this posture and how we can alleviate the pain caused by this?
- What would be the long-term issues with keeping this posture, both emotionally and physically?
- How can we help those with this posture? Which asanas would help?
- How would a backward bend look for someone with kyphosis?
- How do you think an adolescent might have come to have a kyphotic posture?

Some reasons why have a teenager might have kyphosis:

- carrying heavy rucksacks
- asthma or breathing issues
- shyness
- tall
- muscle, fascia or ligament tightness
- low self-esteem
- sitting badly
- screen use.

So, with this group, you need to be extra careful with backward bends, taking it slowly and cautiously.

Exercises to reduce kyphosis

Lying flat on the floor, encouraging shoulders to come down to the floor and lengthening through the back of the neck. Also lying on a bolster, so that it runs along the length of the spine. Some gentle backward bends such as mini-camel can be helpful too.

SCOLIOSIS

Why would an adolescent get scoliosis? When the spine is shaped like an S, looking from behind, there is scoliosis. It is often a little twisted too. It is easy for this condition to go undiagnosed for a lifetime. Although you are not there to diagnose, it might be of interest to know that if you see one hand hang lower than the other (a shoulder lower than the other or a hip lower), when they are standing straight, you are likely to see a scoliotic back. In severe cases you can see a hip or a shoulder higher than the other too.

Some reasons why a teenager might have scoliosis:

- fascia, muscle or ligament tightness
- birth trauma or defect
- general trauma
- carrying something on one hip or shoulder exclusively
- sitting badly for long periods of time.

What can we do to help?

Exercises to reduce scoliosis

For scoliosis, a general yoga practice is ideal, where we are continuously bringing our awareness to alignment, maybe working more on one side than the other, conscious that one side needs strengthening and the other releasing.

Any postures where we have a side-to-side motion or bilateral movement will help. Many students come to yoga specifically to cure their scoliosis. If scoliosis is more than 45–50 degrees, the National Health Service (NHS) will operate a steel rod into the back, to keep it straight, so you might find many students coming to you to straighten in order to avoid the operation.

Back problems – why intervene?

Why is it important to help teenagers with back problems? Because if we manage to intervene at this stage of development, we might stop a trajectory that can lead to chronic and severe pain, not only in the back but also in the legs, shoulders and neck.

Bone density

The bones will become denser when they are under pressure. Can you think of a way in which we might create a denser bone tissue?

Any kind of pressure on the bone will make it denser and stronger. For example, if we jump up and down, the bone in the lower leg and the femur will become stronger in response to the action. Similarly, if we stand on our head, a certain pressure will be placed on the neck area of the spine, which will make it denser and stronger. If we stand on one leg, the bone there becomes stronger – can you think of any other yoga postures and how they might strengthen the bone?

Do you know why bone density would be beneficial for teenagers?

Maybe you are not aware that the bone density of your body as an adolescent determines the density of your body as an adult. There is a definite correlation between bone density and wellness, or rather an adverse relationship between lack of bone density and depression or mental health issues.

A dentist friend of mine once spoke of a mutual friend, saying he feared for her mental health, as she had so many cavities. I asked what he meant and he said that when teeth start to rot it is often due to lack of calcium in the body. When calcium suddenly or gradually dips in the body, it can be due to the brain leaching calcium from the bones or teeth – the brain needs calcium for electrical impulses in the brain. When the brain is overactive, it is usually due to rumination or anxiety. The relationship is also inverse, in that when the bones are depleted of calcium it is an indicator of poor mental health.

Exercises to increase bone density

Standing postures where we are putting pressure on one leg at a time will increase density, as well as arm balances and shoulder stand, all beneficial for bone density.

Athletes and yoga

For many years Sport England have funded yoga as a sport for those who were dropping out of sport. It was seen to be a perfect movement which might keep young people going or maybe even segue them into other sports. This has proven to be true.

Many young athletes are open minded and always looking to become more flexible, more nimble and stronger – yoga is a common tool to achieve these goals. They see it as a tool to up their game! Some examples of athletes who have used yoga both as a sports psychology tool and also to upgrade their physical prowess are: Ryan Giggs (ex-footballer), James Cracknell (ex-Olympic rower), England's rugby and cricket teams, and Jessica Ennis Hill (ex-Olympic heptathlete), to name but a few.

Many athletes work unilaterally – can you think what I might mean by this?

- Tennis players work mostly with what side of their body and which limb?
- Footballers?
- Runners?
- Hockey players?
- Netball players?

You see, there is an unbalance in their fitness, which often causes injury. Several times I have been called in to work with athletes to support healthy growth in the body and heighten their performance through effective and simple strengthening and releasing exercises. Maybe you would like to work out how you would do that with the groups above?

> *I think joining the yoga group has increased...body confidence – she now does a lot more exercise at home...and is proud that she is stronger and fitter. I think before this she didn't think that exercise was 'her thing' because she didn't enjoy team competitive sports. Yoga has played a part in convincing her she can be fit, strong and healthy.* (Year 9 (age 14–15) parent)

Many have come back to me reporting greater nimbleness and less injury. I call yoga preventative physiotherapy – you will find this group of students highly motivated to practise at home, as long as they are given reasons for the intervention. They will practise beyond what you have given them with curiosity and determination.

General exercises for athletes

Focus on the area that is under duress in their particular game (e.g. footballers, focus on the knee, hamstrings and quadriceps; swimmers on shoulders and hips). Also, always look at how you can stretch the muscles and release tension, paying particular attention to any unilateral stretches that might be necessary.

Exercises to treat Osgood Schlatters disease

In young people who play ball sports that involve kicking, there is a high risk of Osgood Schlatters disease, where the kicking action has resulted in an inflammation of the area just below the knee where the tendon from the kneecap attaches to the shinbone. This is a painful condition that often results in stopping playing altogether for at least six weeks, while the inflammation subsides, and the young player needs to practise some very specific exercises to reduce inflammation and bring about healing. These stretches are often the hero pose and other gentle stretches of the muscle just above the knee cap.

Hormonal changes

Menstruation

It has been found that when a young woman reaches the weight of 42kg she is likely to menstruate. Which means, of course, that if there is some kind of eating disorder the natural age for first period will shift either up or down.

Obviously having your first period in many cultures is a very important and celebrated event. It is the moment we transition from girlhood to womanhood. However, for many, periods have become a nuisance or even shameful. We see advertisements with young women running or dancing in white trousers, advertising that you can do anything on your first day of your period, where most of us lie curled up on the sofa stuffing our faces with chocolate, nesting with a hot water bottle.

What has this got to do with yoga?

Uma Dinsmore-Tuli, who has championed women's causes in yoga in the UK and abroad, recognises that 90 per cent of practitioners in the West are in fact women. There are many beautiful practices that bring our awareness to our sacred femininity, to the profound awe and miracle of being able to bring life to the world and how our bodies and our periods are our signature. Many postural and meditation practices bring our awareness to the sacred nature of coming into womanhood and give permission for deep rest and nurturance during this time. Many young women have no idea about how our cycle can inform and inspire us when we are in tune with it – not only our menstruation or moon cycle but also diurnal and seasonal cycles. Understanding the changing energies of these cycles, and what each one is inviting us to do, gives us immense power and insight. You can read more about this in Uma's wonderful book *Yoni Shakti.*[1]

> *[She is] more physically confident as she has become stronger as a result of yoga – particularly body strength. Happy to talk openly about how she is feeling; good and bad.* (Year 8 (age 13–14) parent)

---

1 Dinsmore-Tuli 2014.

Exercises to support healthy menarche

Movements that are slow, deliberate and conscious, favouring circular movements, releasing the hip and lower back area particularly. Constantly encourage women to move within their comfort zone. Legs up the wall, *yoni mudra*[2] during breathing.

Male growth

For many young men the main hormone at play is testosterone, which can play havoc with anger management specifically. With breathing exercises, focusing and some tough physical postures, it is possible to channel this surge in energy and need for risk taking in an optimal way.

In terms of physical changes, the growth in the chest area allows for greater upper body strength, which can be particularly heartening while they are still quite small, and they can easily carry their body weight on their arms in arm balances!

I remember vividly when one young man of 12 came in to class, having taught himself the peacock, and duly balanced on the table! He was the smallest in the class but had managed to master many tricky arm balances. He was also able to enjoy many acroyoga postures (more advanced partner postures), such as plank on plank!

Exercises to support healthy male development

Any arm balances release anger and build pectoral muscles. Hamstring release and hip release in butterfly and downward dog are also necessary. It is beneficial for young men to do partner work in acroyoga, to feel connected and physically support each other.

Transitions from innocence

For many boys the moment when their voice breaks is one of pride and embarrassment in equal measure. The squeaky high-pitched

2 *Yoni mudra* is a hand position of creating a diamond shape by touching thumbs together and forefingers together over the belly button. The palms then rest over the ovaries. *Yoni* means womb in Sanskrit.

crashing down into the desired manly pitch is often the source of comedy and shame. Finally established in the deep voice, however, young men notice a shift in the way others view them. One of my students used to take the public bus regularly to school; sometimes he would forget his money for the bus and the driver would let him in, allowing him to pay the following day or maybe even letting him have the ride for free. One day, after the summer, he forgot his money and the same bus driver chucked him off the bus, miles away from the school, on a country lane. Needless to say, the boy arrived very late for school, drenched and cold, scolded for the second time and it was only 9 am! What had happened? His voice had broken! The bus driver no longer saw a cute young boy but a threatening, manipulative young man. Perceptions of young men in our society have a deep impact on them and many feel hard done by and simply respond in kind, by being the threats that they are expected to be, finding power in this profile which is shoved upon them. Others may vainly try to recover their innocence, through kindness and pathological altruism, with varying degrees of luck.

Similarly, one of my female students who had always cycled to school, oblivious to her surroundings, finds herself being whistled at, jolted suddenly into a sexualised world. All this due to the new body that had developed without her agency. Others had decided that she was now sexually available and aware, even though she herself was not. I remember vividly how shocked and self-conscious she became from that day on. She was sad and unprepared to lose her childhood.

In both these cases, it was other adults who made a judgement on the adolescent – that they are entering a sexualised world, whether they were aware of it or not, whether they were willing participants or not. This brings to mind the statement of the wonderful neuroscience researcher Sarah Jayne Blakemore:

> If we treated old people or toddlers like we treat adolescents, there would be an outrage. We make fun of and look down on teenagers in regular intervals in this country in a way which is bound to render them introverted and insecure.[3]

She is referring to comedian Harry Enfield's Kevin the Teenager character.

3 Blakemore 2015.

Conversely, some can't wait to arrive into adulthood, casting off the world of dolls, trains and dependency. The moment cannot come fast enough, ready to burst out of the home and what is defining them into a new world of possibilities and adventure. Personally, I remember borrowing tampons from my friends, pretending that I had my period, stuffing socks in my bra to look bigger than I was! The moment a boy asked me out was a moment of celebration; the moment I actually got my period I remember shouting out to the whole family and dancing on the table! I felt that finally I would be taken seriously, I would be allowed to make my own decisions and have autonomy. But then when I was asked out and went on dates, I felt clumsy, awkward and ignorant – trying to navigate other people's demands with my own desires and needs.

There is a binary tendency in British society today to demonise or put teens on a pedestal – either they are problematic and criminals in the making or they are victims of crimes. In my mind, if we truly understood that they are in a transitionary phase in their lives where trying things out, that leaving their comfort zone and taking risks is biologically driven behaviour, maybe we would be more patient and understanding, allowing them in turn to take their place and be supported by society at large.

Exercises to help with transition

Encourage inward looking, reflecting on what feels good and what doesn't, exploring their own boundaries when it comes to pleasure and pain and what is OK and what is not. Allowing them to pull back from a posture if it feels too difficult but encouraging them to give it a go – especially arm balances, which provide resources for balance, focus and strength. There may be postures that they could do as children but, due to changes, they can no longer accomplish. Acknowledge these. In relaxation, let go of the expectation of others and feeling into their own needs and letting go of them too eventually, until they are at peace with the ground and those around us.

Sexuality

The most striking element of adolescence is, of course, the burgeoning sexuality heralded by gender-defining physical changes. Breasts in girls, pubic hair and testes dropping in men. The outward signalling of the ability to conceive and create life, the availability and maturity for sexual encounter. For many this is a confusing moment. Can you remember when you started to be aware that you had sexual feelings? Did it come as a surprise or had your friends and family supported you towards that transition? Was it a time to celebrate or a time of shame? Were you ready or did you feel coerced or forced to become sexual? Did your body develop in time with your feelings?

For many, the first sexual feelings, whether attraction to another or simply 'feeling horny', come as somewhat of a surprise. For many young men, their sexuality almost takes over; getting random erections on the bus at 13 is one element that has been described to me. For women in many cultures (most, I would say), any feelings of sexual attraction are often shameful or labelled as 'slutty'.

Today there is the added issue of gender fluidity. This is a controversial topic which has come to our attention in the last few years in the UK, including young people changing their bodies to fit the gender they identify with, through various operations and chemicals. Within this area is obviously also sexuality confusion; as the openness around homosexuality grows, many young people grow up unsure of which gender they are attracted to and many report that there is no such thing as gender – we are all on a spectrum of gender and we are simply attracted to a person, notwithstanding their gender. With a holistic yoga practice, which encourages the witnessing of the breath, the body, the mind, we no longer identify merely with the body, and therefore gender, but with something more nebulous, more majestic and satisfying, which is beyond gender.

Exercises to think about healthy sexuality

Honouring the body, recognising sensations, feelings, emotions and thoughts, knowing where boundaries are and how they feel. What is the difference between like, love and lust? How do I feel them in my body?

Some diseases on the rise among young people

The *lack of bone density*, in other words osteopenia,[4] is on the rise among young people, most probably due partly to lack of vitamin D (the sunshine vitamin) and an increasingly sedentary lifestyle – 'the sitting disease', coupled with increased cases of anorexia nervosa.[5] We need an active approach to combat this problem, which will have a long-term impact on our NHS – can you imagine the impact of young people who have osteopenia on the NHS?

Exercises to improve bone density

Anything where you are putting pressure on a single bone, such as arm balances, shoulder stands and one-legged standing poses.

Obesity is another disease which has doubled in the last ten years among young people.[6] Obesity often leads to diabetes and osteopenia as well as poor muscle tone and depression. It is considered a mental health problem as overeating is a sign that we are trying to cope with emotions that seem out of our control.[7] We must not underestimate the impact of obesity on the whole body, as well as future healthcare costs, and the pressure on joints, the heart, the bones and the digestive and physiological systems. Long term, there is a very high probability that obesity continues into adulthood as eating habits and fat levels are usually set at this time.

Exercises to combat obesity

Vinyasa flows,[8] adapted to limited movement (similar to pregnancy). Be aware that many obese children are also hypermobile, so focus on movement and strengthening rather than flexibility.

Another disease that is creeping down in the ages is *Type 2 diabetes*,[9] often linked to the above; also often considered a mental health

4 Osteopenia3 2018.
5 Guardian 2011.
6 Connolly 2016.
7 Young 2015.
8 *Vinyasa* is a Sanskrit word with many meanings, often used to describe flowing from posture to posture.
9 Alberti *et al.* 2004.

issue due to illogical and unnecessary emotional eating linked to mental states rather than physical need (hunger). It is also linked to chronic stress, as glucose is needed for cortisol to be constantly present in the body, so the body craves sugar, and the pancreas can no longer cope with the amount of insulin it needs to produce and crashes. Long term, this is extremely detrimental to the adult and results in a shorter lifespan, a life of controlling diet and meal timings as well as fainting and weakness.

Exercises for diabetes

With diabetic students, you will need to tell them before you start how strenuous the class is and not vary that from week to week, so that they can regulate their insulin appropriately. Calm the nervous system with breathing exercises. A smooth class in terms of energy expenditure is good. Awareness of the sweetness of life and anything they can bring to mind that has made them feel sweet about themselves or others. Self-massage and tuning into their own needs.

We are finding more cases of *rheumatoid arthritis* among young people too. Rheumatism is understood to be an inflammatory disease, connected to a stress response and lifestyle factors. So again, stress-related diseases that previously dominated in middle age are creeping down to adolescence (juvenile idiopathic arthritis).[10]

Exercises for rheumatoid arthritis

Simple, joint-freeing exercises are helpful as well as anything which reduces stress and anxiety, thereby reducing inflammation in the body.

One of the most worrying issues among young people is *self-harm*, which has risen through the years. In 2014 figures suggested a 70 per cent rise in 10–14-year-olds attending accident and emergency departments for self-harm-related reasons over the preceding

10 Kumar 2010.

two years.[11] Those who self-harm will often say that they do it to 'feel something' or because they feel out of control in every other sphere of their lives and take ownership of their body in this way. Their time is tied up in school work and other activities that are often prescribed for them, so the self-harming becomes an escape. Contrary to common opinion, both boys and girls engage in self-harm.

Exercises for those who self-harm

Self-massage, *metta* meditation,[12] partner work and strong postures, particularly arm balances.

Summary

Our physical growth and maturation bring many welcome and unwelcome shifts which make us almost unrecognisable to acquaintances and relatives and sometimes even to ourselves. These changes can be alienating, making us feel as if we are living in an unwelcome vessel. However, when managed with yoga asana in particular, they can become a source of power and insight. When we sometimes stumble across more or less severe issues (back problems, obesity, osteopenia) they could be adequately and effectively supported by a simple weekly yoga practice, which gives awareness of the changes occurring as well as tools to support both a healthy curiosity and a healthy respect towards a strong and functioning body.

---

11 SelfharmUK 2018.

12 *Metta* meditation is a special meditation which comes from the Buddhist tradition, meaning a loving kindness meditation. It involves repeating loving words and directing them to specific people and towards one's self.

— Chapter 5 —

HOW TEENS EXPERIENCE SOCIETY

Leaving innocence behind

> The backpack from the festival stands by the washing machine. Unrecognisable tickets and objects spill on to the floor. I am not on Instagram, I can't see the photos. The groups he went to see are unknown to me. The friends he went with I have only met fleetingly. As social media offers photos of gingerbread baking seven years ago, it hits me hard that the two boys in my house today are in no way recognisable as those boys in the picture. This boy now has another life, no longer centred around the home. What happened? They stepped into society; they stepped outside their village, their home, their cocooned environment and abandoned themselves to experiences that I had no control over. They started exploring the world outside the home. They started finding out about how and where they belong within this new world.

When did you leave childhood? When did you start to feel like an adult? How did that process evolve? What did you feel you had to do in order to be treated with respect in society and by your peers? Take a few moments to reflect on these questions in your journal.

This chapter will take a look at which challenges young people face and how yoga could help. It is with some trepidation that I delve into this topic, as there are so many different experiences to take into account. The UK has many different social strata; there is a huge discrepancy between wealthy and poor, cultures, religions, urban versus rural, sexual orientation and experience of gender that have their specific issues and problems. They all have varying and sometimes diametrically opposed experiences and the sands are shifting daily in terms of drug culture, social media, school and family. However, here is a generalised overview that can help you to understand the tendencies, if not the endlessly shifting detail, of young people's lives.

School – preparatory or imprisoning?

For many young people, school is central. It is the hub of the drama, the discipline, as well as the source of anxiety. For others, it is the respite from a chaotic home life. For a few, it is impossible. Many young people find school overwhelming and anxiety provoking and have school phobia or cannot cope with the discipline and rigour of school to such a degree that they are excluded from school as a disciplinary measure. They have the impression that schools are prisons, a place they have to be according to the law, where discipline is at the core, which has no real connection to the lives they lead or envisage leading in the future. In an ideal world school would prepare us for the future, a future where we belong with full agency, empowered to make a difference with support from elders who are there to mentor and guide us. Initially in the nineteenth century school was a social experiment, to prepare young people for a life of obedience and compliance in factories and offices. Today, many of those jobs are automated.

What does the future hold? Young people will not be stepping into a tailor-made job market but rather forging their own niche with their specific profile and branding. For this they need vision, empowerment and agency. Does school in the UK encourage this? I would argue it does not. In general, many professionals working in education feel that the British academic system is out of touch and does not address society's needs for a visionary future. In some cases school is a holding station to bring down unemployment figures and separate the academics from the manual workers, and to keep young people off the streets. Several psychologists in CAMHS who I have worked with have said to me that they feel that the school environment is in fact one of the major causes of the rise in anxiety for so many young people. The constant pressure on schools to provide results filters directly down to teachers, tutors and students to simply perform and achieve. They are bound to feel that they are never good enough; every time they reach their academic goals they are given higher goals. The love of learning, the safe community, the curiosity and exploration that form the core to any truly successful learning and teaching experience are lost.

With yoga as part of the school day, teens are encouraged to develop an inner life and release each stressor as it comes along, leading to compassion, which in turn leads to prosocial behaviour. For many, the yoga class is the space where they drop the mask of achiever, best friend, antagonist or protagonist in whatever dramas are unfolding. These dramas include teachers, peers and family, which form a backdrop to their whole emerging identity.

With each step that we take outwards in society to forge our identity and separate ourselves from our family, we need to dive deep inside to check in with ourselves that who we are becoming has integrity and congruency. In this way we can safeguard our mental health by developing our sense of agency, which is such an integral part of wellbeing.

We need to encourage our young people to see themselves as part of the big picture, belonging to their community and intrinsic to the future of the world. In yoga terms this is called *dharma*. As with so many Sanskrit words, the word dharma has many meanings. In this context, we mean our role in life, that upholds the righteous and the good. What are we good at and called upon to do which would benefit humankind in some way? In Simon Haas's beautiful book *The Dharma Code*, he unveils four pillars to your dharma: *ahimsa*, *tapas*, *satya*, *saucha* – non-violence (love), discipline, truth and purity (clarity). When we engage in these 'pillars' we find our path easily and readily.[1]

Take a moment at this stage to journal on these four pillars; if you were to be absolutely truthful with yourself (and others), and thought (and expressed) clearly what you love dearly and dedicated yourself to it with discipline – what would the outcome be?

From a teenager's perspective, it would be interesting for a moment to ask, is this something that our current school system is concerned with? Do schools try to support young people to find

1 Haas 2015.

their path in life, their way to belong in society, where they can make a difference?

Flo, who is 13, says:

> I do yoga because I enjoy having time for myself quietly and I find myself coping much better in every area of school. I think it would be good to have in all schools, in PSHE for example. We are told that mental health issues are very common among us young, but we're not given techniques to support ourselves. Yoga is such a technique.[2]

Peers and friends – litmus testing my emerging character

The role of a teenager is to become an interdependent individual, someone who can be relied upon to take responsibility and receive the privilege of respect as an adult who belongs in the context of society. The people around them determine, to some degree, how they see society, whether they are successful, supported and solid or whether they are a 'failure', maladapted and alone in the world. Any traumatic past will automatically hardwire the brain towards vigilance and heightened wariness around others and potentially simply repeat damaging relationships. If they have never experienced a strong attachment, they will find it harder to trust and build close and strong bonds with others.

They see the world through the lens of what has gone before. In yoga, we call this *samskaras* – the grooves in the mind that we tend to repeat, reacting rather than responding. After all, how we see the world is who we are. When we feel supported and confident we see the world as an optimal place where we belong; conversely, if we find it hard to trust anyone we see the world as a place where no one can be trusted.

Yoga can help with this and change the trajectory of a life by calming the nervous system and creating a trusting environment within school which may allow the teen to develop integrity within themselves which, in turn, allows them to develop stronger and more intimate bonds and healthy relationships with peers as

2 Cross 2017.

well as trusting their own future and the world at large to be a predominantly positive place where they can meet challenges with courage and grace. What a gift!

Sex in society – the game changer

The main difference between the child at primary and at secondary school is the burgeoning sexual desire and the emerging identity that is coloured by that desire. Never has sexuality or gender been as fluid and open as it is in the UK today. For many this liberty has offered empowerment, for others it is confusing and a cause for anxiety. I had a private client who, at 12, mused that he thought he might be gay. On asking him what made him think that, he replied that two boys at school (an all boys' school) had been kind to him following a bullying incident. Their kindness was so overwhelming to him, as he had been an outsider, that he interpreted it as sexual attraction. On the other hand, many of us would not recognise the tolerance and kindness that exists in schools today around gender and sexual preferences. Another pupil of mine told me that when he was 15 one of his friends thought he might be gay so, to help him along, he went with him to a gay club to support him.

Connection through tablets and smartphones has introduced free and copious access to pornography from an early age into every young person's life. Due to the nature of online presence, young people are accessing pornography like never before. Through 3 and 4G, a frightening number of young people, as young as 11, are accessing pornographic sites.[3] Many of them are guided to them through ads on unrelated sites. There is a large range of pornography, ranging from hard core to 'female friendly' porn. In the UK the statistics are staggering:

> About 53 per cent of 11–16-year-olds have seen explicit material online, nearly all of whom (94%) had seen it by 14, the Middlesex University study says. They also discovered that it was more likely for the youngsters to find material accidentally (28%), for example via a pop-up advertisement, than to specifically seek it out (19%). More than three-quarters of the children surveyed – 87 per cent of the boys and 77 per cent of the girls – felt pornography failed to

3 Sellgren 2016. The following quote and statistics are also from this report.

help them understand consent, but most of the boys (53%) and 39 per cent of girls saw it as a realistic depiction of sex.

Some of the children's approach to sex was also informed by pornographic scenes, with more than a third (39%) of the 13–14-year-old and a fifth of the 11–12-year-old boys saying they wanted to copy the behaviour they had seen.

The report also found:

- More boys than girls had viewed online pornography through choice.
- 135 (14%) of the young people who responded had taken naked and/or semi-naked images of themselves, and just over half of these (7% overall) had shared these images.
- Of those children who reported seeing online pornography, the greatest proportion (38%) had first seen it on a portable laptop, 33 per cent through a mobile phone and just under a quarter (24%) on a desktop computer.
- Nearly 60 per cent of the children and young people surveyed who had seen online pornography reported seeing it for the first time at home, followed by 29 per cent who reported doing so at a friend's house.

According to a US review of present statistics:

- Teenagers with frequent exposure to sexual content on TV have a substantially greater likelihood of teenage pregnancy and the likelihood of teen pregnancy was twice as high when the quantity of sexual content exposure within the viewing episodes was high.
- Pornography viewing by teens disorients them during the developmental phase when they have to learn how to handle their sexuality and when they are most vulnerable to uncertainty about their sexual beliefs and moral values.
- A significant relationship also exists among teens between frequent pornography use and feelings of loneliness, including major depression.

- Adolescents exposed to high levels of pornography have lower levels of sexual self-esteem.[4]

The statistics are clear: the more exposure teens get to pornography, the less likely they are to have satisfying sex lives. The expectations from both partners is unrealistic, to such a degree that there is a rise in violence within relationships as this is thought to be 'normal' as depicted in porn films.

An interest in sex and a curiosity about the opposite sex is natural and hormonally driven. However, it is a curious world that floods 11-year-olds with images never to be forgotten of degrading sexual behaviour and violent communication in the realm of sex and intimacy.

Yoga is a practice in radical self-care. When taught correctly, we are continuously being brought back to 'what feels good', 'our heart's desire', 'feeling the body' and 'releasing tension in mind and body'. These practices bring us to a place of agency in our body, where it is no longer possible to disembody ourselves in order to pleasure another, or to *perform* sexuality in a way that does not bring us pleasure. Yoga roots out the problem of pornography, which is that of disconnection, and brings full awareness to our right as humans to connect deeply and meaningfully with another just as we are learning to connect with ourselves.

Family

The transition from child to adult is hugely impacted by the home environment. If home life is chaotic, our attachment bonds to our carers are likely to be chaotic, so it will be difficult to feel supported in our search for positive and interdependent individualisation, away from the family. We might be rejected in our search for a new identity, or maybe we are needed as a carer ourselves in a family, further hampering our ability to search outside for meaning and a new context. However, if our home life is stable and our attachments secure, then we are more likely to be supported in our search for identity and our turning away from the family. The family will always be there to support and scaffold in times of need but will set us free when we are ready.

4 American College of Pediatricians 2016.

According to Bowlby's ground-breaking research, adolescents who had been taken away from their primary caregivers for six months or more during the first five years had a much higher incidence of psychopathological behaviour.[5] This was his '44 thieves study' in 1944, which concluded that 86 per cent of 'affectionless psychopaths' had experienced six months or more of separation from their mother in the first five years. They were characterised by lack of guilt, lack of concern for others and lack of ability to form long-lasting bonds.

His research, and other more recent research papers that focus more on adolescent years,[6] finds that a positive attachment during these years is key to the forming of prosocial identity. It seems clear to me that the ability to trust and be trusted within the family is directly correlated to the ability to engage and take responsibility in society.

The more we are empowered to regulate ourselves, trust ourselves to self-care and work as a necessary cog in the wheel of family life, the more we will feel able to co-regulate with others, recognise our interdependence and take responsibility in society. How we relate to ourselves is bound to be mirrored in how we relate to others and the world around us.

It is wrong to assume that the moment they reject parents or carers, teens are ready to leave. There are plenty of practice runs, followed by falls, where parents come to the rescue to pick them up again. The tension for many parents during this time is beyond anything they have ever coped with before. There is evidence in recent reports that depression among parents can be worse during the teen years than post-partum, due to frictions and difficulties at home. It can be especially hard for single parents to get the balance right between maintaining a strong bond with their children and letting them go. Many times I have witnessed teens leaving home at 16, because the situation had become intolerable for both adult and child. These chaotic home lives can catalyse young people into precociously early sexual relationships.

As Robin, 18, said:

5 Mcleod 2007.

6 Lapsley, Rice and FitzGerald 1990.

> For me, meditation, visualisations and yoga helped with my very difficult relationship with my mum when I was around 14, so that we could get on and understand each other better. I would take a breath, relax and then it would be much easier. I was on the verge of leaving home, but then it got better.[7]

Wider society

Environment/politics

Since primary school children have been made aware of the relationship between themselves and the environment. More than any other generation our young people are acutely aware that the future of our planet is at risk and that they are the ones who will be dealing with it. They have grown up with Earth Day, recycling and learning about the cost of consumerism and factory production on the planet. Many feel personally engaged in supporting positive change. As Robin said at the Instill Conference in 2017:

> For me, yoga was about self-awareness which gives me self-confidence, which affects the relationships with your family (yoga helps you improve your relationships with your parents) – giving self-compassion, to yourself and others, then of course the environment. People our age are worried about the environment, we feel responsible for the damage, we need to make solutions. Yoga is not an obvious solution, but it is, as we become more aware and we can heal our environment through yoga.[8]

I thought this was an insightful comment on the connection, which many see, between sustainable living and yoga.

When we become more aware of how our actions are impacting us, then we become gentler towards everything else, which we realise is part of us, whether it is another human, an animal or the environment (Nature). The deeper our connection is to the world around us, the more respect we feel. A sense of belonging to Nature and our planet is necessary for us to want to protect it. Unfortunately, for many the outside world is just that, outside of awareness and outside of experience. As we spend more time

---

7 Watkins-Davis 2017.

8 Watkins-Davis 2017. The quotes by Robin that follow are also from this source.

indoors than ever before it will necessarily impact our experience of nature and the environment.

Social media

Social media is at the heart of young people's lives. It is a means of communication that plays a central part in identity, trust, friendship and connection. Social media is primarily a tool for connection; it helps shy youngsters get in touch with people they like, it helps them and us connect with friends quickly and easily, literally chatting with people at any time of day or night across the globe. Many young people are consistently taught about social media at school, how to regulate, how to filter fake news and how to protect themselves. We use terms such as 'meet' online, making no distinction between meeting in person or online. Snapchat, Facebook and Twitter are the most popular networking sites, with Snapchat probably having the biggest impact on everyday communication.

It is my impression that, for many young people, social media, as the name suggests, is society. It seems to be a place where they are judged, found, discarded and paraded. It is where they are scorned and praised. It seems to be more real for some than the physical world itself. Moreover, what for many of us would have been unimaginable only a few years ago is that their society includes people who they have never met, from all over the world. However, due to the algorithms of social media, there is a strong tendency towards echo chambers of values and beliefs. This means that, just like small real-life communities, social media supports and echoes our own beliefs and values, potentially making us even less tolerant and understanding of the 'other'. The added element of being able to 'block', 'ghost' or delete someone may give us the false understanding that people are objects to be used and discarded.

Social media has created a bedroom culture, which may impact negatively on the cohesion of the family. The multiplication of devices in the home increases the individualisation within the family, where all members of the family could be watching different films or TV series at the same time, as opposed to the 1970s household, where the family had to negotiate their viewing together around the television set. So outside influence entered the living room in the 1950s with the TV and is now entering uncensored into each and every bedroom.[9] What this means, in fact, is that risk for young people is no longer out on the street, where they spend on average less time than prison inmates,[10] but in the confines of their own bedrooms. Conversely, the impression among many parents is that outdoors is not safe, and that is why the children are kept indoors.[11] This move towards the bedroom as the mainstay for adolescents is part of that individualisation and can also have the impact of eroding cohesion in the family.

Our society has become increasingly individualised; your social media account knows almost everything about you, from your political leanings to your friendship circles and interests; your Netflix account knows what you want to watch; your Spotify account knows your taste in music; your shopping account knows the food you like.

The commonly held perceptions about social media seem to indicate that social media is predominantly a pernicious player in the lives of teens; however, the jury is out, as research continues to come in that may give us a clearer picture in a few years' time.

How much true connection are we actually gaining through social media? And what impact does this have on our young people? What is your experience?

When we asked Rebecca about social media she said: 'I like social media, I meet lots of other yogis and connect with them on social media, it's good for me.'[12]

Gabe, 17, on the other hand, said: 'I find it degrades my attention span; when I do yoga, it forces you to redirect your attention to yourself, refresh yourself.'[13]

Edie, 16, said: 'A big factor in anxiety for young people is the social media, according to research – through doing the yoga, it detaches you from it. Yoga enters every aspect of your life. I don't take my phone out, I hardly ever have it on me now. It helps you be detached. It can be so addictive.'[14]

---

9 Livingstone 2002.
10 Carrington 2016.
11 Carrington 2016.
12 Dion 2017. The quote by Rebecca in the next section is also from this source.
13 Watts 2017. The quote by Gabe in the next section is also from this source.
14 Bainbridge 2017.

We will expand on this crucial and central topic later on in these pages, looking at the impact of social media on isolation, loneliness, bullying, body image and how yoga can support young people to engage with the internet in a healthy way.

Stereotypes and yoga

Many people ask: what do young people think of yoga? What are the preconceptions?

It is clear that many young people have the impression that yoga is a predominantly older female sport, which is true. Some say it is even unmanly! However, two young men spoke about this at the Instill Conference in 2017; the first said:

> Yoga should be for everyone, it's not about performance, not for athletes or women – it's for everyone. (Gabe, 17-year-old A-level student with no sports interest)

Gabe had been struggling with anxiety and, when his art project went wrong, he found himself having a meltdown. He decided to start going to yoga and found it had profound effects on his anxiety levels. He uses a technique where you focus on a light or a point in the room to bring your mind into one-pointed awareness. He taught the delegates at the Instill Conference to practise this technique.

The second young man said:

> The other guys in the rugby team thought I was weird when I suggested yoga, but then they realised they are doing it already as part of their warm up and cool down, so that was cool and easy to bring in more after that, especially as they realise the benefit. (Asher, 16, rugby player)[15]

Asher had suffered from anger issues and been to see an anger management therapist, who pointed him towards yoga. The simple breathing technique of breathing in for three and out for six, then extending the breathing for a few minutes, had an immediate effect and meant that he did not have as many issues with anger, which made a big difference in his life.

---

15 Watts 2017. The quote from Asher in the next section is also from this source.

Robin, the leader of Team Bliss (a group of young people in the UK who all feel that yoga is an essential part of the school curriculum, based on their own experiences of how it helped them in their lives), underlined that it can be off-putting for a young person to come to a yoga class, as it is usually full of older people, and that needed to be addressed:

> Most of us feel that yoga is for older people like our parents and grandparents, so when I came along to teach, it was good 'cos then younger people could come too, 'cos not everyone is comfortable in a class full of grannies! (Robin)

Rebecca had become severely ill and was confined to a bed with wasting muscles for several months when she was only 14. Determined to get stronger, she took up yoga. She overcame the preconception that yoga was just for able-bodied athletic people and used it as a kind of physiotherapy to build up the wasted muscles. She now teaches acroyoga to teens! She is particularly keen to let people know that she 'bases' in acroyoga, which means she can support anyone on top of her in the postures; this involves a significant amount of physical and mental strength.

Flo, a 16-year-old student at an all-girls school, did a survey at her school and found young people had various responses: 'a weird exercise', 'a way to connect to god', 'a hippy thing', 'a spiritual thing', 'I don't know'. When asked if they would consider going to a yoga class, 50 per cent said maybe and only 15 per cent said no.

Definitions of yoga included:

> The movement of your breath and body, a way of finding connection, finding yourself, finding connection with people. (Rebecca)

> A way of understanding myself and my body. (Asher)

> Moving the body, relaxing and breathing and then show them. (Robin)

The dark night of the soul

> *As a young teen, I wondered why so many of us lived in a state of restless dissatisfaction with life. I hoped I might find a mentor, an example to follow; but wherever I looked I saw people struggling*

with the same basic challenges: jealousy, anger, frustration, boredom, dissatisfaction. I was no exception of course. A witness to the difficulties experienced by loved ones, I questioned Western culture's response to crises and where our perspectives might be failing us.

Simon Haas, *Yoga and the Dark Night of the Soul*, 2018[16]

When we birth ourselves into society with the fresh eyes of a teenager, we have clarity, we see fake, we sense anomalies, we rage against injustice, we feel deeply and hurt painfully and soar in ecstasy. We seem to vibrate with full vitality. Our brains are renewed, they have the enormous potential to recreate themselves; in this extremely malleable state there seems to be an urgency to understand, to see through the bullshit and to take a stance. These qualities tend to become an intrinsic part of this transitional time and form a part of most teenagers' character. These feelings of urgency, delight and exploration are the very essence of vitality.

As Haas so eloquently states, the objectives and goals presented to young people in society often leave them feeling lost and dissatisfied, which is why, I believe, yoga has become such a popular pastime for so many. Yoga has a rich secular philosophy which can support young people, in particular, by giving answers to some of the trickiest existential questions arising from emerging into such a materialist society as ours.

Most young people are bound to question the meaning of life as they start to rise above the parapet of home and look outside. For many, it is a tricky and overstimulated existence they find themselves in, without a clear trajectory, a bigger picture or a belief system. Many take refuge in earning money as soon as they can to go shopping on a Saturday and fill their wardrobes with the latest fashion, which is becoming increasingly cut price and throwaway. They spend their time taking care of their looks and making sure they are as attractive as they can be for the selfies and carefully constructing the life that they want others to see on Instagram.

The natural existential angst becomes heightened by the vigilance of FOMO (fear of missing out) as they fall asleep at night with the phone on their pillow. Instead of spending time building

16 Haas 2018.

an inner world, all their energy is spent looking outwards, building their brand of themselves.

Yoga is such a perfect antidote to this outward-looking stance. We can offer solace in the inward-looking nature of yoga, held softly in the safe embrace of a gentle yoga class: a non-competitive space, where we are encouraged to find room for radical self-care and a unique value system that engages us and supports us in our longing to belong to a rich, deep and meaningful existence, that of our own divinity or universal consciousness.

'How I have benefited from yoga classes'

> Yoga has had many positive effects on me both mentally and physically and none more noticeable than on my patience; both the concentration required during the more complex phases of the asana, as well as the focus required to clear my mind during the relaxation period, has succeeded in ameliorating my ability to focus for an extended period. Miss Pindoria's ability to cater for the less able students (of which I am one) has meant that students of all levels of strength and flexibility are able to practise to their full potential.
>
> Having not been expecting to enjoy yoga it has pleasantly shocked me. The difficulty and serenity of the postures has required me to engage my core and mind. Holding a posture is inextricably linked to focusing and breathing. In this sense, yoga has enabled me to become more aware of my body. (Dylan Kaposi, L6 (aged 16–17), Haberdashers' Aske's School)

> Having never done any form of yoga before, my opinions on it have changed drastically since my first session in November. Being oblivious as to what yoga is about meant that I would never have started it on my own account until I had the opportunity to do so through our Enrichment & Enhancement sessions every Monday.
>
> In the midst of our stressful lives both in and out of school, I think yoga is the key to finding a way to cope with the world around us. After a week goes by, I look forward to the next session to start off the hectic week ahead, by clearing the mind and engaging fully with my body, forgetting those around me. I feel a sense of calmness that helps me at the start of the week. Obviously with

yoga come the physical benefits such as strength, flexibility and stamina, but over these weeks I think I have valued yoga more for the effect it has had mentally. Following the sessions, I feel much more awake, being able to engage more and heightening my level of concentration during class time.

As there are no worries of what the others think of you in the sessions, I feel the postures which we carry out regularly provide me with a positive challenge in a non-competitive environment. I have tried my hardest at reaching the more difficult postures, even when an easier posture has been taught to us. Even though someone else may be doing it and I want to reach their level, these yoga sessions have taught me to push myself to see what I can and can't achieve, reaching the limits of my own ability. This is a skill which can be transferred outside the yoga classroom as well.

I have appreciated the time set aside in my timetable for these yoga sessions in the past weeks and I hope that yoga can be introduced more into school life, so that others can understand the benefits of it. I will indeed find a way to continue yoga even after this rotation comes to an end, as there is so much I want to learn and there is no other way, that I could think of, to better my wellbeing. (Animesh Misra, L6, Haberdashers' Aske's School)

Gang culture

Young people come together in groups, it is the natural phenomenon that precedes pairing off into couples. The values and purpose of the groups differ and vary according to social status, religion, area and gender.

Gang culture fulfils the needs of young people because there is a clearly defined hierarchy and sense of belonging and codes of conduct. They exist in many different contexts, and have been a way to survive financially and socially in deprived neighbourhoods around the world for centuries. One could argue that there are 'gangs' in all walks of life; in the upper echelons of society, we call them the Freemasons, fraternities or clubs! In deprived areas, they often involve ethnicity, drugs or religion. There is an unspoken code of conduct that is adhered to in order to belong – they are often male; you will be alienated and thrown out if you don't adhere to the unspoken laws, which are often beyond draconian.

Radicalisation

My students in Muslim countries and cultures are deeply concerned about the rise in radicalisation in the UK and abroad. Islam, at its heart, is a peaceful religion, encouraging tolerance and kindness. The terrorist acts supported by a small group have killed, maimed and hurt many people and damaged the reputation of their religion and impacted on their day-to-day life, resulting in rife Islamophobia in certain parts of the UK and the USA. In schools across the country teachers are given guidelines on how to recognise and identify youth at risk of being radicalised. Radicalisation is a process by which a person or group comes to adopt increasingly extreme political, social or religious ideals and aspirations that undermine contemporary ideas and expressions of the nation. Many fear that radicalisation leads to terrorist attacks and therefore danger to the general population, as was experienced in London and Manchester in 2017.

Remember the main drivers of young people? Belonging to a group, connecting with others, taking risks and finding meaning. These are fulfilled in extremist contexts, where ideals and aspirations, a sense of making a difference-to-the future, are paramount and defining. It is not surprising that it is relatively easy to attract young people to this kind of movement. Through history young people have always wanted to make a difference and have their voice heard. It is up to us as elders to guide them towards a healthy way to belong and take risks.

— Chapter 6 —

HOW DOES YOGA HELP YOUNG PEOPLE?

Charlie bounces in, yoga mat in hand – early, often dragging a less-than-willing friend into the common room. They play fight, crashing about, bashing each other over the heads with yoga mats, rolling themselves up in 'sausage rolls' until they finally manage to settle down and shake off the day, ready for the yoga. He is a well-balanced, fun, intelligent guy who is on the A team for rugby, hockey and cricket. In the beginning he comes with various injuries, a broken collarbone, a torn ligament, stretched hamstring, bruised pride. He states clearly that his intention is to up his game. Slowly he is injuring himself less and less. One day he is a little quiet; when we do our check-in at the beginning of the class, he mutters: 'Mum has been away for a week now, she's with my uncle and I think she should come home.' We pause. As a group, we knew Charlie wasn't OK. We waited. 'I miss her, my uncle is sick, he might die, but I want her to come home.' He fell silent. We sat quietly for a while. Then we began a silent, slow and strong practice, which allowed his tears to fall gently; we ended with a group tackle/hug. When a psychologist came to research the group a few weeks later, Charlie told her that yoga always changes his mood and it makes him feel more connected to everyone around him, even the people who aren't in the room. Charlie will always live on in my memory as I plan classes for young men; he taught me about their need for showing vulnerability and their need for being safely held in a non-judgemental space.

Stress as imbalance

Stress is the experience of being under pressure. It is a natural phenomenon and the word comes from physics – the stress on a certain material causes it to break or strengthen. In similar ways, if we are resilient, stress makes us stronger. If the amount of stress we receive is within our coping zone, we manage to become more resilient. However, if the stress is above and beyond what we can cope with, we break under the pressure, becoming either mentally or physically sick.

Young people have a pretty stressful existence – sociologically, physically and neurologically. Anthropologically, many cultures had severe and gruelling rites of passage for their young people to prove that they were ready for adult life and to support the transition to prepare them for adulthood. However, long-term (chronic) stress lies at the base for many different kinds of illnesses, such as obesity, diabetes, inflammatory diseases and depression – even schizophrenia and Alzheimer's disease may be triggered by stress.

> *I'm more confident in school and in PE and am more energetic – I am less stressed at school and I can deal with things better. I do yoga because I usually get stressed, anxious and achey and yoga feels as if those things are no longer there. My favourite is the child pose.* (Holly, 13)

Initially stress causes the mind to speed up, able to make decisions quickly and almost intuitively – we call this the flow state. When we are in eustress (beneficial stress, a stressor which makes you more resilient and leads to personal growth; it is met with vigour and hope), we move quickly, effortlessly, using the correct amount of energy to quickly and effectively immerse ourselves fully in the task at hand with full joy and awareness. When we are in this eustress state, we feel like we are capturing the moment, riding the wave, with not too much rumination, lobbing the ball right back each time it comes towards us. This flow state is considered to be the optimal state for humans to reach – no rumination, no anxiety, enough going on for us to feel stimulated and awake, but not so much as to make us anxious and exhausted. We can exist in this flow state indefinitely, the body responding in a relaxed and effective manner to everything that comes our way. We are fully at ease.

In yoga, we call this state *sattwa* – harmonious, pure state, balanced, we are in contact with our intuition. When you dance with another you are in the flow state together, moving in harmony, reading each other with utmost presence. Some relationships are like this too, where we are harmoniously connecting every moment, without compromising ourselves. This state is our optimal human state, which most of us call happiness or presence. Everything we do is an attempt to come back to this state.

What takes us out of this state is imbalance – too much stimulation (whether physical, auditory or mental – the food we eat, the environment around us, the music we listen to, the books we read, the company we keep, sudden events beyond our coping zone, too much exercise and so on; we call this *rajas*) or too little stimulation (whether physical, mental or through the senses – laziness and lethargy, food and drink that brings us down such as alcohol and pre-cooked food, too little exercise; we call this *tamas*).

Once we are out of balance and back into *tamas* or *rajas*, we tend to go into a seesaw motion. In order to bring ourselves out of *tamas* we exaggerate our *rajas* – and then, to come down, we veg out and go into *tamas* again, never quite finding the sweet spot of *sattwa*. As we come out of balance, the body seizes up, becomes stiff and tense, or the opposite, in *tamas,* when it becomes lax and lacks muscle tone completely, growing old before its time in both scenarios.

The mind becomes overwhelmed and either races ahead in a *rajas*ic anxious fervour or lags behind in *tamas*, looking backwards in depression, guilt and shame. Both of these have chemical indicators – in anxiety, there is a lack of GABA, lack of dopamine and an overproduction of cortisol. In depression, the most common neuro-correlates seem to indicate a dip in serotonin levels and in prefrontal cortex (PFC) activity after a prolonged period of hyper-excitability in the amygdala region, often resulting in a smaller hippocampus. According to all research yoga boosts serotonin, GABA and dopamine, while down-regulating the amygdala and cortisol production, so reversing the neurological status of these two conditions.[1]

---

1 Uebelacker 2010.

The autonomic nervous system

The body's autonomic nervous system is made up of the parasympathetic and the sympathetic nervous systems, described simply in the following infographic.

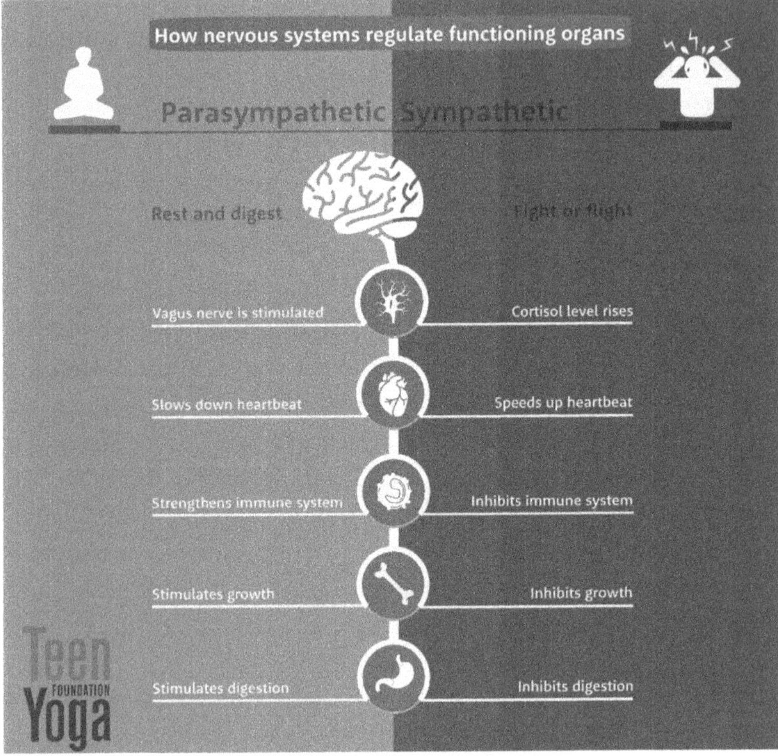

Let's focus for a minute on the importance of balance, *sattwa* and, in particular, hormonal balance in the body. The autonomic nervous system is divided into two parts – the sympathetic and the parasympathetic system.

When the body is in stress, our sympathetic system takes over and allows us to respond quickly and effectively. This is a useful and helpful response when we are in danger or angry. As long as we can come back into our parasympathetic system, we will be back in balance (known as homeostasis). In any kind of trauma or PTSD (post-traumatic stress disorder) the sympathetic system has become hardwired to stay engaged and vigilant. This has a long-term impact on the brain and the body. If your body is constantly pumped full of adrenaline there are a few very specific results:

- you will need more glucose to create cortisol (crave sugar → weight gain → obesity and diabetes)
- your amygdala will be overexcited → sleeplessness → low mood → arguments with friends → antisocial behaviour → fall in academic results
- your hippocampus will shrink → harder to retain information and harder to learn
- your PFC will remain underdeveloped → less executive function → getting into trouble → antisocial behaviour
- adrenal fatigue → exhaustion, ME, chronic fatigue
- pancreatic fatigue → Type 2 diabetes
- digestive issues → irritable bowel syndrome (IBS), diarrhoea, constipation
- tense muscles → back pain, neck pain, shoulder pain, joint stiffness, long-term pain and inflammation
- reduced immune system → more general sickness, time off school, lethargy
- inflammation → rheumatism, arthritis, stomach ulcers, colitis and so on
- respiratory issues → asthma
- impeded growth as all the nutrients are basically used up by the fight or flight mechanism and there is little left for growth.

As you will see from the diagram, when the parasympathetic system is in charge the body tends to focus on the following activities:

- rest
- digesting food
- balancing hormones
- breathing deeper and more calmly
- growing well
- boosting immune system
- combating inflammation

- creating homeostasis in the body.

So it is important to understand, then, that the body craves to be in balance, able to swiftly move from sympathetic to parasympathetic at a moment's notice, much like a herd of horses suddenly aware of danger, who gallop to the end of the field together at a switch of the tail, only to dip their heads and eat a moment later. It is not desirable to stay in parasympathetic, or we become *tamas*ic and unfeeling robots, who fail to connect with the world. Nor is it desirable to be constantly switched on, with our minds and bodies racing at 100 miles per hour in the *rajas*ic mode. We need to learn to come into balance – into *sattwa* – and we do this by tuning into Nature, our first teacher, honouring the rhythms of the day, the week, the month and seasons of the year.

When we stimulate the vagus nerve in various *yogasana*,[2] it elicits a parasympathetic response, where the heartbeat slows down, the immune system is strengthened and growth is boosted. Digestion also benefits from the parasympathetic nervous system. Earlier in this chapter we covered how stress works in the body, which is the machinations of the sympathetic nervous system – helping us to run away or fight, it speeds up the heartbeat, injects cortisol into the bloodstream, and inhibits digestion, growth and immunity, among many other factors.

Particularly in deep breathing and in backward bends, the vagus nerve is stimulated and, according to Stephen Porges's polyvagal theory,[3] then elicits the parasympathetic response. If you cast your mind back to a time when you felt anxious, you will notice how your heart beat faster, so, conversely, when our heart beats more slowly it will always be comforting and supportive, bringing us into harmony.

A study on how teens feel about yoga

In a research paper we conducted with Leeds University,[4] we invited a small group of young people to discuss with a researcher

2 *Yogasana* is a Sanskrit word meaning a steady pose to create union. It is used as a synonym to *asana*.

3 Porges 2001.

4 A. Morgan 2013.

how yoga made them feel. The researcher came once a week over a three-month period to create a qualitative research paper. It was a rigorous and robust piece of research, although small, with only 15 participants. Here you will see the main themes that were raised during their discussions:

- greater social cohesion
- more effective pain management
- ability to shift states (mood)
- greater autonomy over personal achievement
- greater agency and autonomy
- greater willingness to commit.

Some are more obvious than others – we know that our mood will change after a yoga class. But, for young people, this is such an empowerment: to know that if I feel a certain way, I could feel completely different if I do some yoga. Imagine the long-term effects of this act of agency! Currently, when people feel low or stressed, they may reach for a parent, a friend or, worse, the bottle or the pills. If at an early age they learn that they can use certain tools to change their mood quickly and effectively, it would change the trajectory of their lives for the better. Also, pain management is powerful, as this is the age group where we start to have autonomy over our medication, and if we start habits of regulating pain through movement rather than drugs it may well create a healthy pattern for later in life. I love the social cohesion – this meant that everyone in the group felt better about everyone around them after their yoga session, whether they knew them or not. Basically, their relationship with the world had shifted. To be committed to something and achieve change is the basis for any growth mindset tool and can easily be translated to other areas of our lives, such as academia and friendship. Autonomy and agency are, as stated earlier, the main tasks of adolescence; and if the yoga class is giving them the feeling of autonomy and it is something they want to come back to, then we are supporting healthy adolescence, which is probably the most important consideration. Take a look at the summary of this research in the following graphic.

'You can be the person that you like to be in yoga'
How young people explain the benefits of yoga

Amy Morgan
Institute of Psychological Sciences, University of Leeds

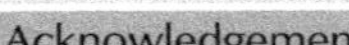

Introduction

- Research has shown that the number of young people reporting feelings of depression and anxiety is rising (Collishaw et al, 2010) and there is a trend for the rates of these disorders to increase in the transition between childhood and adolescence (Costello et al, 2011).
- There is a growing interest in positive psychology (Seligman & Csikszentmihalyi, 2000) which focuses on positive human development, leading to a more preventative as opposed to reactive approach to mental illness.
- Various studies have shown that practices such as yoga, meditation and mindfulness have a wide range of benefits, including effectiveness in decreasing levels of depression and anxiety (Bonura & Tenenbaum, 2013; Pilkington et al, 2005; Woolery et al, 2004).
- However, most of this research has been done in adults and the majority of research done in children has used quantitative approaches, limiting our understanding of the extent to which it's helping children as well as how aware they are of its effects.
- This current study uses qualitative approaches in order to try and get a deeper insight into how young people explain the benefits of yoga.

Method

- 10 participants voluntarily involved in the yoga classes (8 female, 2 male, age range=11–13 years)
- Had attended the yoga classes between a month and a year, some had previous experience
- Recruited through the yoga instructor to take part in the study
- Information letters and consent forms given to the participants, parents and head teacher of the school
- Each participant took part in a semi-structured interview which was recorded and transcribed
- Transcripts were analysed using thematic analysis in order to find common themes in the data

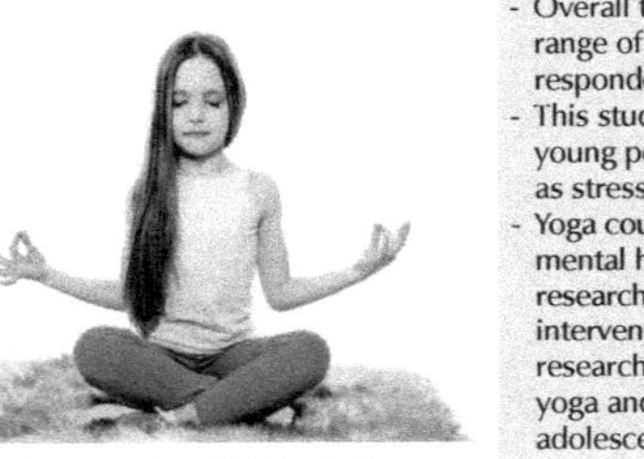
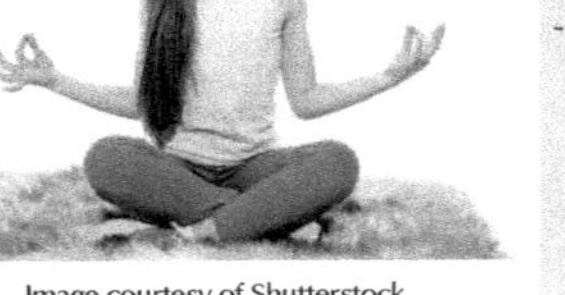

Image courtesy of Shutterstock

Analysis

1. Shifting in state from before the yoga class (stressed state) compared to after the yoga class (calm state)
2. Measurable self-improvement, which led to an increase in confidence and self-esteem
3. Sense of freedom and independence with a lack of judgement
4. Sense of commitment; using self-discipline and dedication; had to keep attending the yoga class in order to reap the long-term benefits
5. Feeling more connected and developing a greater understanding of others
6. Enhanced sports performance and active approach to pain

Conclusion

- Overall the young people were able to articulate a range of benefits of the yoga classes and responded positively to it being taught in school
- This study gives a greater insight into the needs of young people and how negative influences, such as stress and external pressures, can be reduced
- Yoga could be an effective prevention of poor mental health, but there is need for further research into the feasibility of this kind of intervention in schools, as well as longitudinal research to investigate the long-term benefits of yoga and mindfulness in childhood through to adolescence and adulthood

Number of participants reporting themes

Number of participants
10
9
8
7
6
5
4
3
2
1
0

Shifting states
Personal achievement
Autonomy
Commitment
Social cohesion
Sports performance and active approach to pain

Themes

References

- Bonura, K. B., & Tenenbaum, G. (2013). Effects of yoga on psychological health in older adults. Journal of Physical Activity and Health, 11, 7, 1334–1341.
- Collishaw, S., Maughan, B., Natarajan, L., & Pickles, A. (2010). Trends in adolescent emotional problems in England: A comparison of two national cohorts twenty years apart. Journal of Child Psychology and Psychiatry, 51, 885–894.
- Costello, E. J., Copeland, W., & Angold, A. (2011). Trends in psychopathology across the adolescent years: What changes when children become adolescents, and when adolescents become adults? Journal of Child Psychology and Psychiatry, 52, 1015–1025.
- Pilkington, K., Kirkwood, G., Rampes, H., & Richardson, J. (2005). Yoga for depression: The research evidence. Journal of Affective Disorders, 89, 13–24.
- Seligman, M. E. P., & Csikszentmihalyi, M. (2000). Positive psychology: An introduction. American Psychologist, 55, 5–14.
- Woolery, A., Myers, H., Sternlieb, B., & Zeltzer, L. (2004). A yoga intervention for young adults with elevated symptoms of depression. Alternative Therapies in Health and Medicine, 10, 60–63.

Acknowledgements

Thank you to Dr Siobhan Hugh-Jones and Charlotta Martinus for helping with this research

In any study the teacher (in this case me) is instrumental in how the children perceive yoga and what they gain from the class. We can never divorce the practice from the teacher.

The classes were conducted in a common room as an after-school club for 11–13-year-olds. I normally start by simply asking them how they feel today and asking them what they think yoga is. Then we go through a simple *vinyasa*, usually the sun salutation. I am constantly looking at how I can give them more autonomy, by letting them demonstrate or teach a part of the class or decide what is going to be in the class. By lesson 3 they get the *savasana;*[5] from then on we can take longer *savasana,* and by lesson 5 we can start doing partner poses, if there is a good feeling in the room. By lesson 6 they have a basic understanding of how the various exercises affect them and have started practising at home. By lesson 7 I am starting to introduce various breathing techniques, all the while checking in with them and making sure we are supporting their needs and responding to stuff that is happening in their lives – meeting them where they are!

There is a small body of research on the results of yoga practice. The research is very clear on the impact of yoga for young people; we have also been collecting anecdotal evidence over the years, all of which clearly signals the massive impact yoga is having on thousands of young people across the UK and beyond. The prevalent themes are: pain management, coping better with exam stress, academic work and friendship issues, managing better at home with issues in the family, and also clarity in how to manage emotion and mood more effectively.

> *Yoga makes me feel comfortable and calm within myself. It makes me feel happy, energised and refreshed and ready for the days ahead. I feel more confident and able, which means that I concentrate and cope better in school.* (Olivia, 13)

Confidence is a theme which I love to see in these quotes, often indicating that the teacher is uplifting in their verbal cues, supporting students' choices in the classroom and optimistic in their outlook.

5 *Savasana* is a Sanskrit word meaning corpse pose, which is traditionally used at the end of a yoga class to help relax the student.

I find it particularly interesting to hear about the parents' perspective, who reiterate this confidence theme – bringing in body confidence as well as intellectual and cognitive confidence.

> 'It relaxes me so I feel like I am almost floating.'
>
> 'It makes you feel refreshed and calmer after a hard working day.'
>
> 'When I can't sleep, I use the relaxation and breathing exercises to help, and after I play tennis I often do yoga stretches and poses to make sure my muscles don't ache.'
>
> 'Relaxed, sleepy, happy.'
>
> '...like my problems don't matter.'

Feeling deeply relaxed is often an outcome of yoga and is usually due to the combination of some strong postures, followed by a deep relaxation.

Calmness and confidence are the themes of these quotes; the yoga seems to bring about relief and courage for young people, which is translated into other areas of their lives. It is also interesting to note that confident and calm comes together. Maybe, when we are frazzled, we are unable to focus and so we lose confidence, as we can't understand or remember what is being asked of us.

Research on yoga and young people

The body of research on yoga for young people has come primarily out of two institutes, the Harvard Medical College with Dr Sat Bir Khalsa at the helm and the Patanjali Institute in Northern India with Dr Shirley Telles. Primary issues have been that of sheer volume of size and variety. Many studies only study small groups of 10–30 participants. The sessions are varied in content and delivery, depending on a multitude of factors, such as teacher, environment, time of day, yoga tradition, age group and, of course, content of the course. However, notwithstanding these provisos, there are a few clear outcomes if we review all research over the last 50 years – and this is a relatively comprehensive list of outcomes that have been reported on several occasions, from different yoga classes to different groups in different scenarios. We also have to go with anecdotal evidence from my own teaching of around 100 young people a week for a 15-year period and then another 30 or so adult students, as well as my own 20-year practice. These benefits have been universal and are outlined in this marvellous infographic originated by Dr Sat Bir Khalsa.

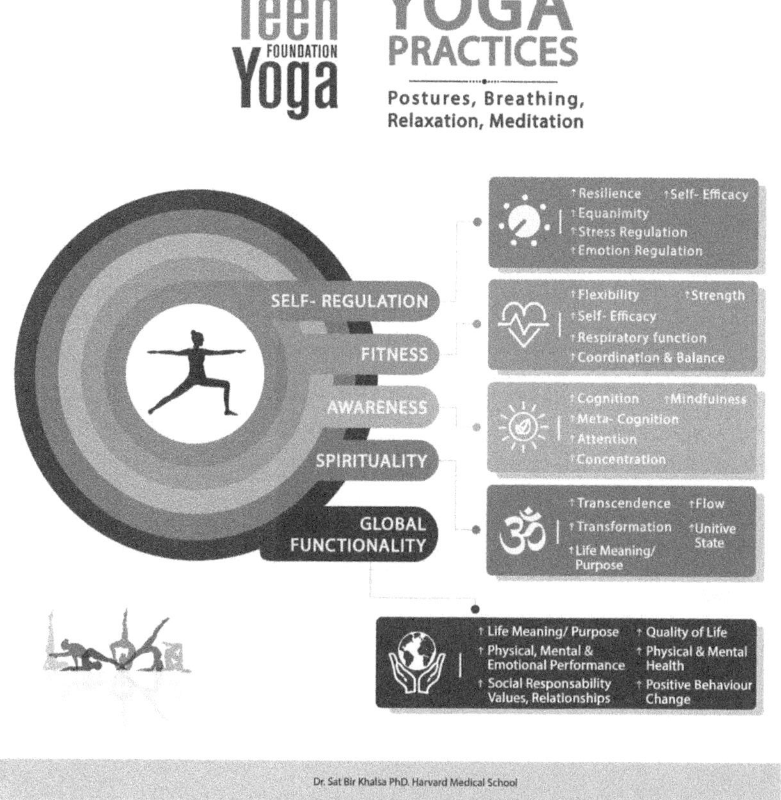

The physical benefits

- Lower blood sugar levels, by calming the nervous system.
- Improved balance, through balancing postures and alternate nostril breathing.

- Relief from chronic pain, through awareness of how to relieve pain through movement and also how to relate to pain differently through mental exercises.
- Anxiety relief, through calming the nervous system by using breathing techniques and releasing tension in the body.
- Improved lung capacity: deep breathing exercises on a daily basis release tension in the muscles around the lungs but also literally expand the tissue of the lungs.
- Relief from menstrual cramps, through various movements focusing on the pelvic area, releasing tension in the muscle groups in the area of the ovaries.
- Lower blood pressure, through relaxing the body.
- Increased flexibility, through stretching fascia and muscle tissue.
- Alter gene expression: Dr Elizabeth Blackburn won the Nobel Prize for her research on how meditation changes epigenetic expression.[6]
- Lower stress levels, through relaxation exercises.
- Improved brain function (more on this later), specifically through alternate nostril breathing but also through calming the amygdala activation and bringing awareness to thoughts, so developing further the PFC.
- Lower risk of heart disease, through cardiovascular exercise.
- Healthy weight, through gentle movement.
- Stronger bones (greater bone density), through placing weight on arms and single legs in balances.
- Greater awareness of the bodily needs and imbalances (useful in avoiding disease), through increased meta-cognition, encouraged by teacher cues.

---

6 Epigenetic expression: inherited genetics, which means how genes are expressed from generation to generation.

- Homeostasis (balance of hormones and rhythms in the body, also in relation to Nature), through learning how to engage the parasympathetic nervous system and down-regulate the sympathetic nervous system.

> *After [yoga] I feel at peace and can work calmly. It makes my muscles feel new at school – I'm always looking forward to yoga. Yoga teaches me not to fight with my siblings. I feel more grounded and I also like learning about my body. My favourite pose is crow because it strengthens my arms and legs.* (Annabelle, 11)

The mental benefits

- Encourages beneficial circadian rhythms, coming in tune with rhythms of the day, the month and the year.
- Better quality sleep, learning how to come into the parasympathetic nervous system through various techniques, when needed.
- Authentic relationships: connecting more deeply within ourselves, we also connect more satisfying relationships with others.
- Increased self-efficacy: with meta-cognition and learning how to watch thoughts and the mind we also learn how to control our expression.
- Increased emotional resilience: learning to see things from a different perspective, where we are no longer at the centre of our drama, we can witness interactions in a more effective way.
- Increased compassion, patience and understanding: through developing compassion for ourselves, we also become kinder to others.
- Regulation of stress, through breathing and exercises specifically designed for this.
- Cognition: activating and expanding the impact of PFC activity through conscious breathing.

- Mindfulness, as part of the eight-part procedure of yoga – the eight limbs include three limbs that are directly connected to mindfulness: *pranayama*, *pratyahara*, *dharana*.
- Meta-cognition: coming into the witness state.
- Attention: becoming aware of thoughts helps us bring attention wilfully.
- Concentration: focus comes with emotional regulation.

The spiritual benefits

- Transcendence: by managing the body and the mind we learn to transcend them.
- Flow state: making just the right amount of effort to feel in the flow.
- Transformation: changing the way we see ourselves and others through control of the mind and body.
- Unitive state: feeling connection with others around us through breathing and moving together in harmony, in trust and compassion.
- Life meaning and purpose, through gentle, guided and compassionate introspection.

Research conducted over the past 30 years on yoga and young people has shown some clear and continuous outcomes, borne out by the great work in the Research Review of Butzer and Dr Khalsa, patron of the TeenYoga Foundation.[7] There are clear specific medical and psychological outcomes which we can state and claim with confidence. But, in the main, what is the overarching result of yoga, which we are keen to share with our young people? When anxiety and depression are as prevalent as they are, we need to teach young people how to use their bodies to ground themselves and also connect with each other.

The findings from a 2016 review make a good summary to remember:[8]

---

7 Khalsa and Butzer 2016.
8 Butzer *et al.* 2016, p.22.

> Research suggests that providing yoga within the school curriculum may be an effective way to help students develop self-regulation, mind–body awareness and physical fitness, which may, in turn, foster additional SEL [social emotional learning] competencies and positive student limitations/implications... Given that research on school-based yoga is in its infancy, most existing studies are preliminary and are of low to moderate methodological quality... yoga could become a well-accepted component of school curricula. It will be particularly important for future research to examine possibilities around integrating school-based yoga and meditation with SEL progams at the individual, group and school-wide levels.

Dr Dan Siegel and David Rock, patrons of the TeenYoga Foundation, speak of the seven essentials for optimal mental health and I have always felt that they form the core of a good yoga class.

Seven essential mental activities for optimal health

I was overjoyed to come across Dr Dan Siegel and David Rock's seven essential activities for mental health which seemed to chime directly with what yoga has to offer young people.[9] Using the body to ground us and connecting with our breath, we find solace from our chattering, wandering mind. This infographic goes into more detail on how exactly this is achieved, and below I have outlined how yoga achieves these seven essential activities.

This infographic is useful as an aide-memoire for optimal mental health. It states the seven essentials for optimal mental health:

Sleep – being the most important, without this we have no energy to lift ourselves up, to be positive or to think straight! In yoga, we support healthy sleep with an increasing *savasana* through the weeks leading to a possible yoga *nidra*.

Connecting – with others in a meaningful and deep way, which makes us feel supported and needed by others. We do this initially by making the students aware of how to connect with themselves, leading on to connection with others within the class and later with others within the community.

9 Siegel 2011.

Time in – being by oneself, reflecting, journalling, meditation. This is an aspect which we try to support, leading the student towards an introspective state.

Play – making life fun and playing in a yoga class is essential, not only so that we can learn but also so that the students want to come back.

Physical – some kind of physical activity is always important for the mind and body – postures will always do this.

Focus – working or having an objective that brings us pleasure and meaning. If we do not focus, we are likely to fall over in certain balancing poses.

Downtime – proper relaxation – which is what we do at the end of the class.

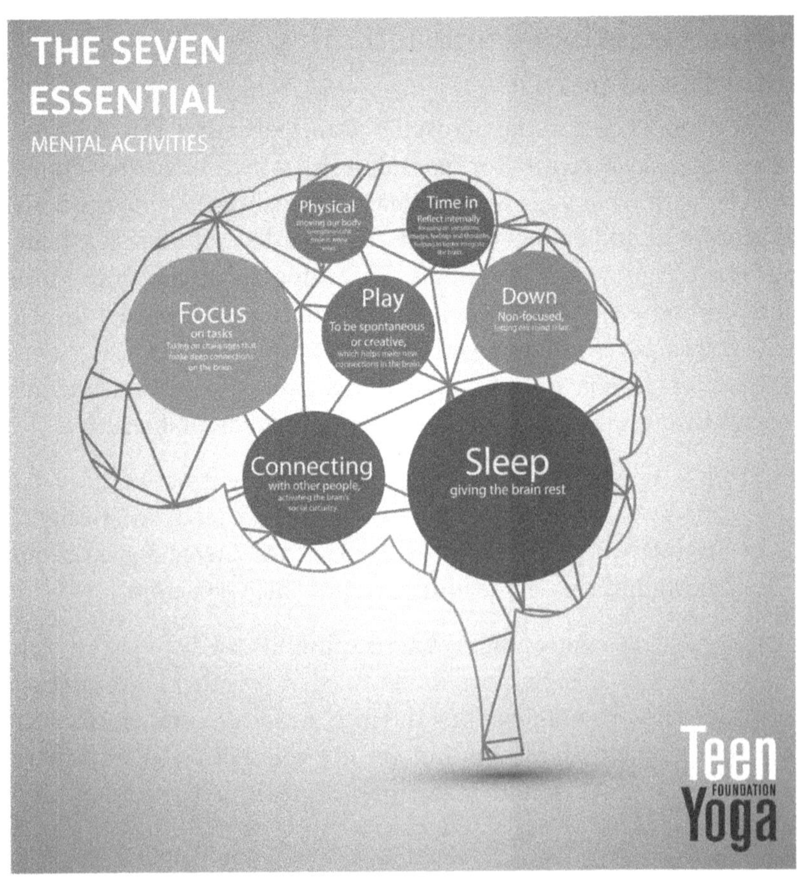

So, for me, these became the seven pointers for a great yoga class.

- We know that most young people suffer from sleep deprivation; according to studies most sleep on average seven hours per night instead of the recommended nine hours.[10]
- Connection today is something that needs to be learned, as we increasingly spend time on screens and slowly our addiction turns us away from connecting properly with others. On average, young people spend up to five hours per day on screens,[11] affecting their sleep patterns, social connections and social skills as well as mental health.[12]
- One of my students, a psychiatrist, said, when asked, that being alone was the scariest thing for most young people – being away from connectivity and others. However, spending time by oneself is the time we give ourselves to reflect, journal, touch base; this forms an essential part of shaping our identity, clarifying what is important and connecting with our conscience. If we don't know how we feel on the inside, how can we express who we are and what we want? There needs to be a fluid relationship between inner experience and outer expression, which can only happen if we spend time quietly. When we are congruent, we feel at ease, knowing that what we are expressing is who we are and what we want, rather than what is expected of us. We need to encourage reflection, in order to develop integrity, congruency as well as optimal independence, interdependence and emotional regulation.
- Playing gives joy and vitality and connects us with others and ourselves in the best possible way – in yoga, we can do this by introducing partner poses and acroyoga.
- Most yoga classes are physical; our bodies are made to move, so lymph and blood can easily move around the body and the muscles can stretch and flex, in order that the teenage body

10 Bradford 2018.
11 Weston 2017.
12 Jenkins 2017.

can grow with ease and manage spurts and transitions more pleasantly, and boost the immune system as well as help with sleep. There is some evidence also that certain postures and visualisations may support healthy hormone balancing, which clearly is an important aspect while they are shifting so dramatically.[13]

- In order for us to achieve anything in life, focus is needed, whether it is to learn to drive a car or to be there for a friend. In yoga we tend to focus during balancing postures particularly.
- At the end of the class and after particularly tricky postures, give them a nice long *savasana*, where they get to properly relax. The body scan must be the most effective tool of yoga; when given after a moderate workout and breathing practice, you are offering both your mind and body a complete reset. If young people learn this as a coping mechanism to overwhelm, then maybe they might avoid alcohol or drugs, which are the most common coping mechanisms in our society and are embodied and modelled by parents and adults. This has much deeper and more long-lasting effects than many of us can imagine.

How might you design a class with these seven elements in mind? Take a moment to journal a few class ideas, bringing into mind the seven essentials.

The eight limbs of yoga and a yoga class

In summary, yoga has the ability to bring our body and mind back into balance, in various ways, particularly in an integral and complete approach to yoga, including all the eight limbs:

Yamas – ways we relate to the world

Niyamas – ways we relate to our self

Asana – steady postures, proper exercise

13 Rodrigues 2018.

Pranayama – breathing techniques to steady the mind, using our breath to find optimal health and balance

Pratyahara – looking inwards, time in

Dhyana – focus

Dharana – meditation, one-pointed focus to lift ourselves up

Samadhi – bliss

There are some very striking similarities between Dr Dan Siegel and David Rock's infographic and the eight limbs. Yoga becomes such an incredibly rich and diverse modality to really engage, embrace and empower young people. If you, as a yoga teacher, have all these tools at your fingertips at any given moment, you will be well equipped to support young people.

Yamas and *niyamas* could be translated as connecting with the outside world in an ethical and correct way. Asana is exercise. *Pranayama* is an essential tool to reduce stress and a bridge to the time in. *Pratyahara* is time in, *dhyana* is focus and *dharana* is connection with the divine aspect of ourselves. *Samadhi* can be the ultimate joyful and blissful state.

I suggest that we use the *yamas* and *niyamas* as a way to empower young people to find their moral compass and to attune themselves to the society they live in. You can use them as themes for your classes, so teaching asana while imparting the philosophy.

Each yoga class would ideally take these eight limbs into consideration and perhaps work through them. Too many teachers see their job as a gym instructor, busting shapes that impress and are fun. The purpose of this book is to remind us all that yoga is so much broader than this and can support our young in many other ways. When we move into the breath work, I tend to focus on Brahmari[14] and three-part breath to begin with – immediately we are teaching 'time in', a moment of reflection and stillness in their busy lives. This segue into *pratyahara* is the moment when most of us get hooked on yoga and forms the basis for any meditation practice in the future. As one of my main teachers,

14 Brahmari is also known as humming breath and constitutes simply covering your ears and eyes while humming out loud as long as the breath continues and then taking a breath and starting again.

Swami Sivadasananda, said in a film I made – '*Pratyahara* is our segue into the inner world, the beautiful, blissful state, which once experienced becomes our internal resting place which we will always long for.'

There is another way to look at it, a useful dimension which is less known. The *pratyahara* state will teach each student the beauty of introspection and sitting for a moment in the flower of your own heart, the power of focus and also that inward focus naturally leads to concentration (as we are less aware of outward distraction) – the tool which is so important for success in any sphere of life which naturally leads to the blissful state we call *samadhi*.

Another approach which works with young people as a therapeutic tool is to work with the five bodies. The *koshas* in yoga are:

Physical body – *annamaya kosha*

Breath body – *pranayama kosha*

Mind body – *manomaya kosha*

Wisdom/intuition body – *vijnanamaya kosha*

Bliss body – *anandamaya kosha*

These are a wonderful representation of all our capacities as a human, going deeper and deeper into more and more subtle realms of our 'humanness'. Initially we believe, feel and see that we are only the physical body, but for many this is dissatisfying and frustrating, especially within the yoga world. For many young people it is the way into yoga, as this is the way it is described – 'how to get the yoga body!' We will never be slim enough, strong enough, tall enough. Coming into the breath is a relief from this obsessive thinking and can calm the mind down and is a direct connection to the mind, allowing our focus to go inwards (*pratyahara*) – immediately we focus on our breathing and shift it, we notice a subtle shift in our minds. So now we can identify with other aspects of ourselves, taking the focus away from the physical and more onto 'How do I relate to the physical?' – a kind of meta-perspective that can alleviate our struggles. Once we are observing the mind, we can see its machinations – '*I always think about this, when I am with her*' or '*Isn't it interesting how my mind is lifted when I go to yoga!'*; we start to understand the subtle cues that the mind takes to go down various routes, thus giving us an insight in how we might be able to shape our thinking for the better. If we are invited into stillness by our teacher, it is also possible to go beyond the chattering, unstable mind and into a quieter, more subtle form of knowing, beyond intellect and logic and where there is wisdom. This is the place that truly believes that everything is for the best. This is a deep place of ease and *sattwa*. We see every situation or experience as an opportunity to learn and grow. We 'know' what to do in various circumstances as we start to trust the universe to guide and nurture us. When we are truly in this place, we come to a place of bliss and equanimity which initially might be a little precarious, but eventually forms part of our character. Imagine how this might impact someone who is growing up, their demeanour, their attitude towards life, expectations, friendships, work and society at large?

What is your experience with the five bodies – have you ever had any insight into the benefit of stilling the mind? Have you ever noticed intuition coming to the fore in moments of insight?

The practice of yoga teaching

It's all very well, you having amazing lesson plans and an insight in yoga and even an insight into the situation of young people in the UK today, but if you don't know how to bring it forward and actually share it appropriately to their group, then what is the point? Some of you might be teaching groups, others in one-to-one scenarios – either way I thought this infographic might be of some use, as it is highly accurate and compiled by some pupils at one of the best schools in the country. Maybe they are the best precisely because they listen to their students?

How to be a good teacher

This is the infographic that the Crossley Heath School in the UK (one of the top schools in the UK at the time of the research) made about how the teacher might approach the students in order to get the best results.

Teen Foundation Yoga

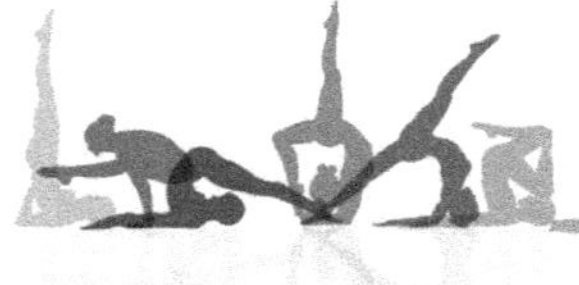

7. Control of Class

6. Motivation & High Expectations

5. Encouragement and Praise

4. Clear subject knowledge/varied teaching styles & resources

3. Passion and Enthusiasm for the subject

2. Sense of Humour/Fun

1. Approachability/Care/Support/Empathy/Help

The Crossley Heath School hierarchy of students' preferred teacher behaviour

Before we can even get in the door, there needs to be a sense of humour and fun rolled together with care, support and help. These qualities are hard to feel and share when we are stressed and tense, which is why they have become such valuable currency.

To be passionate about one's topic is always good for you and the student as enthusiasm is often contagious and encourages engagement.

To be encouraging is more important than making their posture or attitude right – you are much more likely to get the group on your side if you are praising and sandwich any criticisms within the praise.

When we expect great things of our students, they want to please and fulfil our hopes for them, they try harder and you motivate them with your expectations. My mother was a teacher for around 50 years and her students always got the highest marks in her subject. I know that she truly loved them, she encouraged them, she saw their strengths and weaknesses, she supported them and stood by their side. She is still in touch with many students, decades later.

It is interesting to see that control of class came at the top of the triangle on two accounts, first as it is a direct result of the other issues we have discussed, but also because it means that it is the least important aspect for the students.

Summary

At a time of great change, when body and mind are being primed for socialisation (i.e. moving out of the family home and functioning and adapting to society), young people are calling out for tools to manage the transition. There is a heightened awareness these days that mental health difficulties are on the rise and everyone knows someone who is struggling. In many contexts the use of mindfulness may have paved the way for yoga to be accepted in their sphere. In the UK 'yoga' was one of the most searched for words on Google in 2016, while the yoga and pilates business brings in £812 million a year and rising.[15]

---

15 Delaney 2017.

Commonly, yoga is offered either as an intervention for those struggling with stress, as an enrichment activity or as a physical education (PE) option. It takes over where mindfulness leaves off. It brings in the whole school, whole person (mind and body) approach, priming the individual to be at ease with themselves physically, socially and mentally in order to function optimally in society.

— Chapter 7 —

MINDFULNESS AND YOGA

> Confused, she often burst in, late, dishevelled, noisy and angry. It was her way. They had invited a yoga teacher to come to the school. She went to sit next to Maisie. They giggled, messed about and fell over in the postures, creating hell for the other 30 people in the yoga class. It was part of PE and she never liked PE, but she did like Maisie and it seemed Maisie liked her! When the yoga teacher said lie down, they lay down, held hands and breathed at the rhythm she counted, feeling everything that was going on in the body after the exercises, which had been fun; it felt like dancing, messing about together. Now they were quiet, for the first time, well, ever. She felt her heart beating and her hand was warm in Maisie's hand. She noticed all her emotions, so many emotions, anger at her dad, frustration at her teachers, love for Maisie and calm after a pretty tough workout. It was good to recognise all the thoughts and feelings as they popped up. She no longer needed to express, the agitation had gone. Just for a moment she was peaceful. She would come back.

I remember this student, although it was probably ten years ago now. She was well known for being one of the most disruptive students in the school. The yoga gave her permission to play, then to connect with herself and her friend; she felt she belonged in the silence, when nothing was being asked of her. She returned every week until the end of term. She would stay after class, chatting about yoga, about stuff that was going on for her, about the teachers she disliked. I felt privileged to be part of her world, to be the confidante to someone who was so disconnected and disengaged from school.

Mindfulness in schools

Many schools contact us requiring mindfulness teachers. There is a common perception that yoga is related to mindfulness. What is your impression of how much of your yoga practice involves mindfulness practice? Are you aware of the impact of this dimension in your yoga? How important is it? In this chapter I will attempt to touch on the relationship between the two and how yoga practitioners can learn from the pitfalls of the recent mindfulness movement in schools. Anecdotal evidence from pupils and teachers in schools and university researchers shows that young people are finding mindfulness boring. Maybe it is because most mindfulness classes are seated? Students who sit for eight hours at school, then sit on a bus home, after which they sit to study and even to play games, have a sedentary disease. Their physical agitation, often rooted in emotional discomfort, is not addressed adequately when seated.

In many cases mindfulness classes are not necessarily being offered by mindfulness practitioners, raising issues of authenticity and accuracy of practice. In some cases it seems to be used as a tool to manage behaviour directly (*sit down, close your eyes quietly and breathe, notice emotions, sensations and feelings*) rather than to manage, express and regulate emotion (*I wonder how you are feeling today and how you can acknowledge, express and shift that mood in a healthy and simple way with the movement of the breath and the body*). Similarly, yoga is being offered in gyms and schools by those who have no direct yoga practice or knowledge. When we offer these practices stripped of their majesty, we fail to connect with young people and we fail to meet their deepest desire, which is to find meaning in life and establish their role in society. Let's take a look at what we can learn from the pitfalls of the mindfulness movement and see how it might be possible to nurture the true majesty of yoga in order to serve young people more deeply.

Introduction to mindfulness

The common definition of mindfulness is being present for whatever is, with kindness and without judgement. Some prefer to call it heartfulness! It is a beautiful practice which aims to bring us closer to accepting and finally integrating uncomfortable feelings, memories, experiences and sensations both in ourselves and others. There is an impressive body of research proving that this practice creates greater resilience, self-regulation and co-regulation even among those with depression and PTSD.[1]

Relatively new on the scene, mindfulness has seeped into practically every sphere of UK society over the last ten years. It has been heralded in the UK and the USA as an effective intervention for stress and depression, with the introduction of the MBSR (Mindfulness Based Stress Reduction) Programme offered within the NHS in all areas of the UK for free. The results have been impressive, and the programmes have changed many lives for the better. It is exciting that state-funded institutions are introducing a holistic approach such as mindfulness for mental health to such a large part of our community.

Jon Kabat-Zinn, the US East Coast psychotherapist who brought mindfulness to the West as a stress reduction technique (MBSR), was invited to speak at the House of Commons about mindfulness in 2017, where he stated that the UK had witnessed the greatest success rate in the world in bringing mindfulness into society. He also mentioned that he had always considered mindfulness to be fully effective only when combined with the physical aspects of yoga.[2] However, in the rollout in the UK this key aspect has in the main been missed.

Mindfulness classes have been running successfully in the UK parliament now for many years. When speaking with them about the provision of mindfulness, parliamentarians say they feel comfortable engaging together in a practice that has no religious or spiritual significance. I believe much of its success lies in the fact that mindfulness is perceived to be an acceptable way to regulate and calm the nervous system of people from all backgrounds and faiths. It is a palatable practice that can be adopted by all faiths, genders, ages and populations throughout our diverse culture, addressing the main cause (stress) of so many chronic diseases in our country in an effective, empowering and affordable way.

1 D. Morgan 2010.
2 Kabat-Zinn 2005.

Pitfalls of creating yoga and mindfulness programmes

Having worked within the NHS as a yoga therapist for mental health for many years, I see a problem with creating 'programmes'. Clearly, for research purposes, it is important that what is being delivered is similar in the various contexts, so that results can be measured accurately. Furthermore, it is essential that schools, parents and healthcare professionals alike are on board with whatever is being delivered; this is more easily achieved if it is a replicable programme. However, when we place the student/client/service user/patient at the centre of our focus, which we must, we soon realise that a large part of the healing process lies in a tailored approach as opposed to the programmed, cookie-cutter approach. When we tailor each session to meet the needs of individuals in a group, we inevitably change the lesson plan to ensure full engagement (engagement is the key element to good teaching and therapeutic intervention). As therapists, we all recognise the importance of feeling heard and seen as part of the road to recovery. How can this happen if what is being delivered is not responsive to each individual? In any group you may have some students with anxiety and others with depression, for example. Differentiating the lesson to reach both these types of students is essential in any class and can only occur when we trust the teacher and therapist to deliver what each student needs. For this purpose, yoga and mindfulness therapists need to be given as much autonomy as possible to deliver the appropriate therapy much in the same way as a counsellor would.

We are not always aware of the individual's state of mind when we are asking them to come to stillness and focus. For many, for example those who have been or are experiencing trauma or any kind of difficulty, coming into their mind can be a frightening and unwelcome experience, which may even exacerbate their condition. In yoga we may come to stillness eventually (some never do); guided over a long period, the asanas give us clues as to whether the mind is coming to stillness or whether there are unwanted thoughts and racing emotions (if the body cannot hold an asana, if the breath cannot calm, then the mind cannot still) – so we take several steps to notice whether the student is ready for this experience. It is hard for most of us to be quiet with ourselves.

When we finally notice that the breath is calm, the asana is steady, then we might consider inviting an introspection. This safeguards the student from focusing on any unwanted activity in the mind. When the mind is quiet, and we are still, we tend to focus more acutely on whatever the mind is dwelling on, so as therapists and teachers, we need to be assured that the experience is more or less positive before we guide them into stillness. This is why we need to be cautious about delivering programmes in schools and, instead, err on the side of a therapeutic or tailored approach to each scenario, which is only possible when the therapist or teacher is highly skilled and trained.

Dr Dan Siegel, in his lecture for the TeenYoga course, refers to research where teachers who have a personal practice (which was never shared with the students) had a more profound impact on students than the class where the programme was being rolled out by those who did not practise. I conclude that the integrity and lifestyle choices that go with a personal yoga and mindfulness practice are bound to have more of an impact on the student than any practices that are taught in isolation. We learn by emulation, not necessarily simply by listening.

In summary I would like to see yoga and mindfulness in schools delivered by practising teachers and therapists, who are able to draw on many different tools to meet each individual exactly where they are and offer them a tailored toolbox for their lives to support and guide them through their own specific challenges. Yoga needs to be grounded in the body of the practitioner and connecting with the needs of the students, thereby meeting their needs. When we meet their needs, we have engagement.

Retaining authenticity, being connected and grounded

The missing elements of mindfulness – physical and spiritual

A programmed practice, divorced from its other components and divorced from the students, has much less value than it would if taken in conjunction with other Buddhist practices. When distilling mindfulness out of Buddhism, what has been lost?

Jon Kabat-Zinn had to clean the mindfulness practice of any religious or spiritual connotations, so that it would be more accepted in US culture. Similarly, in order to simplify and maybe make the practice more accessible to all situations and people, the physical aspect has also been lost.

Our mind is not the only component involved in a mental health issue. How can we divorce our mind from our body, from our beliefs or even from our society at large? We are part of a bigger picture which needs to be acknowledged. Maybe rather than isolating mental health issues into the lowest common denominator – the brain – we might be wise to go the other way and look at the whole picture, society, physical, mental, emotional and spiritual. Maybe it is time to look at the entire way of life in order to understand how to get to the very root of the issue.

Which elements of yoga are mindfulness?

If we add the missing elements to mindfulness, namely the social, the physical, the emotional and the spiritual, we end up with yoga in its true sense. Yoga devoid of mindfulness is available in many gyms around the country, with personal trainers and aerobics instructors offering it as an option, without necessarily having any knowledge of the breadth and depth of the majesty of yoga. There is a tendency, which is understandable but which we need to be wary of, to secularise – yoga becoming solely a physical practice and mindfulness solely a mind practice. Both these extremes leave out two essential components, namely the social and the spiritual. As we have learned from the previous chapters, these two elements lie at the heart of teen development – driving them forwards towards adulthood. When they understand how to function in society and find meaning in their lives, they can start on their adult journey. The connection found in spiritual practice and the grounding in finding a role in society fulfil their deepest needs at this time and are their main drivers.

When we offer yoga to teenagers, it is most beneficial if we offer all the elements, which honours their full experience of life. If we offer mindless yoga which focuses only on the physical aspects, we are in fact exacerbating the very issues we are trying to help (dysmorphia, eating disorders, self-harm, social isolation).

If we offer mindfulness divorced of movement we are missing the importance of supporting young people's physical and mental health through physical practice (the bottom-up approach).

Becoming mindful in our asana practice brings the dimension of awareness. When we are guided to be aware of the breath, the thoughts, the body moving in space, we learn to have some distance to our experience. When we distance ourselves from our experience and are able to witness it – any struggles, pain or pleasure, we have more agency and gain the potential to change our reaction and response. This is known as meta-cognition and is something that Sat Bir Khalsa of Harvard University has written about in some depth.[3]

Spirituality and yoga

How can we believe that our mental health has no correlation as to whether we move our body, whether we are integrated in society or whether we have an optimistic life view?

When we work holistically we leave no stone unturned. We address all aspects of being human, moving away from this tendency to categorise, compartmentalise and differentiate one aspect of our humanness from another, mistakenly trying to tie changes down to simple chemical formulae.

We live in a very open and extraordinarily multicultural society, which by its nature embraces all creeds, belief systems and ritual. Spirituality lies at the heart of our country and is even written in the Ofsted outline for good practice in schools – 'Every school needs to look to the spiritual, moral, social and cultural development of each child.'[4]

So we can embrace this essential part of wellness and allow young people to explore for themselves meaning making and connection through various embedded questions (not answers) in yoga.

3 Khalsa 2016.

4 Department for Education 2014.

Summary

Mindfulness is a new, well-researched and well-marketed practice which has had inroads in almost all walks of life in the UK and the USA. You are just as likely to find mindfulness classes at a care home as at a nursery school. Yoga, similarly, has over time found its way into care homes, nurseries, schools and CAMHS. However, it has witnessed a slow burn, initially being introduced to curious imperialists at the end of the eighteenth century and initially delivered to the UK in its philosophical form. Yoga was then introduced to a small but enthralled public in the UK, through writers such as Brunton and Isherwood in the 1930s and 40s,[5] who popularised the philosophy of yoga with their curiosity and sincere searching. The physical practice of yoga came to Britain in the 1960s and has been growing year on year, most recently in an exponential manner. It is reckoned by Dr Sat Bir Khalsa that approximately 7 per cent of the British population now practise yoga with a further 25 per cent of adults keen to try and 50 per cent of adolescents open to giving it a go.[6]

Unprogrammed and free, focusing on individual needs, yoga, in true style, has permeated European culture for over two centuries, influencing philosophers and psychologists such as Freud, Jung and Maslow in clear and obvious ways.[7]

Yoga itself has not survived unscathed through the centuries but rather transmogrifies in order to appeal and apply to the current climate. The impact of yoga on culture and society has been slow and steady, natural and organic, diametrically opposed to the mindfulness wave.

Therefore, we need to learn from the mistakes and pitfalls that the mindfulness movement has come across, such as lack of movement, lack of holistic approach, and lack of grounding and connection with its own roots and in some cases with the young people themselves.

---

5 Brunton 1934; Isherwood 1949.

6 S. B. Khalsa, Yoga in the UK, House of Commons, interview with Charlotta Martinus, December 2017.

7 *Freud and Yoga: Two Philosophies of Mind Compared* (2014) by Hellfried Krusche, Jung's work and Maslow's hierarchy of needs all show influence of the philosophy of yoga, interpreted to suit Western minds at the turn of the nineteenth century.

As yoga becomes more popular in schools and as an individual therapy, we need to honour it as the wide and profound science it is within our culture and offer a natural follow-on from mindfulness, filling the gaps and taking us deeper into radical self-care. When we embrace yoga in its entirety we are more likely to be successful than if we simply extract one element from it and discard the rest. All yoga practices work in harmony and suit different people at different times of their lives or function as a step-by-step approach.

Scaled back to asana, yoga is simply gymnastics, as some prominent researchers in the field are currently positing,[8] and has nothing more to add to the curriculum or culture of the UK. Yoga in its entirety has the added benefits of awareness, witnessing, meta-cognition, optimistic philosophical outlook, breathing practice and relaxation.

Where possible, the yoga therapist needs to be at liberty to deliver yoga in its entirety, so it can function as a complete, holistic and continuous healing modality and lifestyle, which encompasses all elements of being human – appealing to the physical, mental, emotional, community and spiritual needs of our being. In my view this is the power of yoga and lies at the very roots of its majesty, longevity and success.

8 Singleton 2010.

PART II

— Chapter 8 —

THE BODY

For your journal

What is your relationship with your body?

Has yoga changed your relationship with your body?

Do you find yourself judging yourself or others by the body?

What do you think the relationship is between the body and the breath?

It was one night out with friends, I got dressed in my skinny jeans that had once been tight-fitting and now hung off me. When my aunty saw me she went ballistic, and it was when I sent my friend a picture of my outfit and when I barely recognised myself in the mirror that I realised I needed to put weight on. This was April – my first-year exams were in May, but how could I revise and study when all I could think about was food? I hated food. I didn't want to eat food. Food was the enemy. But simultaneously, I had to eat. I had to put weight on. I had to stop bingeing and purging. And so, I made the most difficult decision I have ever made – to put my health first, as something mental had become very much physical.

Three weeks before my exam, I dropped out of uni. I was free. It was a relief. I put everything into self-care and giving myself freedom. But I felt like a failure, I made excuses as to why I was going home so much, why I wasn't at all my lectures...

Eight months on and days after my last yoga session I cannot say that I am free, but I am back to a good weight, my relationship with food is more or less healed and I am more aware than ever of the importance of putting your health first.

> Nothing is worth your happiness. Mental health is just as important as physical health. Eating disorders are not a lifestyle choice but rather a stolen lifestyle by a cruel bully in your mind. (Naomi)

Faddy diets, focusing on the scales, how often we eat, how we exercise, are all results of a body-focused and body-driven society, where we perceive the body:

- as 'me'
- as something to be controlled in order to enhance our worthiness
- as a tool to be bartered with (the better body I have, the more attractive I will be to a more valuable 'other')
- as a reflection of status and standing in society
- as a statement of wealth and health.

I love the allegory of the body as the carriage, the emotions the horses, the mind the driver and the passenger the soul. The carriage is connected to the horses with strong pieces of wood (the breath), the driver is connected with the horses with the reins (*prana*) and the passenger with the driver with the voice (intuition). The connection becomes more and more subtle. But we need to listen to the passenger in order to know where we must go. We need to take care of the carriage, so it can carry the soul and move forward. I have found this allegory from the Katha Upanishad to be most useful in placing the body in relation to other aspects of 'me'. It is sometimes said that the body is a reflection of the mind and soul, as it expresses our blockages and our concerns (see chakra meditation in Chapter 20).

Obesity as a mental health issue

Eating more than the body requires leads to obesity. When we do this, it is often understood to be a mental health issue, such as coping with pain of some sort, whether loss, isolation, grief, chaos or low mood. The food can be used as a muffle to numb pain. More concretely, it can be because we are not getting the nutrients that we need, so the body is craving more, often sweet, foods. It is also clear that psychotropic drugs and antidepressants have a marked impact on weight gain.

Mental health professionals suggest that professionals support obese people to build self-esteem,[1] as there is often a vicious cycle of low self-esteem leading to more eating, which in turn leads to weight gain. Once there is self-esteem in place, obese individuals are more likely to want to lose weight and care for themselves and their bodies.

> We have been considering whole school wellbeing at Kingswood for some time and considering various ways in which we might support the whole school community in taking care of their physical and mental health.
>
> Various initiatives have arisen from this, with yoga classes being one particular example that has really engaged both staff and students. We have had incredibly positive feedback from staff, who say that practising yoga releases the tension in body and mind and teaches them techniques which they can use in day-to-day situations to help them manage better at particularly busy times in the school term. A number of staff have now trained as yoga teachers and this, in turn, is allowing us to roll out a programme to support the students. (Simon Morris, headmaster, Kingswood School, Bath)

Body issues

Dysmorphia

It is not surprising, with the advent of selfies, that there is a growing obsession with body shape. I look at the only photo ever taken of my great grandmother, dating back to the turn of the nineteenth century, and wonder what her relationship with her body was – strong farmers in voluminous dresses, covering most of the body all the time. Compare this to today's young people, whose gift to their potential lover can be a naked selfie or even a dismembered photo of their penis, vagina or breasts. We are encouraged to see our bodies as a random sequence of separate parts that need to

---

1 Devlin, Yanovski and Wilson 2000.

be 'targeted' by specific exercises in order to look as they should. When the body does not look like the body in the magazine or on the social media, which, of course, has been airbrushed and treated, then we punish it with diets or fasting. This is happening across both genders.

Bulimia and anorexia nervosa

The complex and life-threatening eating disorders that become so prevalent in adolescence seem impossible to reach and treat. For many of us, young people with these conditions are way too delicate and tricky to start to support. However, for those of us who may have some experience in this realm, it might be of interest to find out more on how we can support them. For many there is some trauma or wrong thinking that starts off the process, whether it is bullying, low self-esteem, desire to fit in, sexual or physical abuse or other causes. Around 75 per cent of women attending rehabilitation for the condition reported a traumatic event that triggered the condition.[2] This is in accordance with my personal experience of students.

Bulimia is overeating and then purging. Anorexia nervosa is starving, sometimes to the point of death. This can also include overexercising to make sure weight is lost.

Eating more or less than we need is a form of self-sabotage. We are damaging our body, often because of some imbalance in our mind and emotions. So, using the allegory above, maybe the breath (being the link between the body and the mind) is a way in to shift this relationship, calming the mind through calming breath.

Self-harm

It breaks my heart when I see young people self-sabotaging, whether it is eating too much or too little, force vomiting or self-harming with cutting. There are many ways to self-harm and it is a wide topic. Over the last five years there has been a rise in self-harming among young people. Usually this is a case of cutting the arms until they bleed. I have come across teens of both genders

2 Scheel 2018.

who do this, either as a habitual release or as a one-off experiment. Last week, my private client, a boy of 13, came in with a red line along the inside of his left arm, where he had tried to cut himself with a key at school after a bullying incident during class. When we opened up about the incident, he tried to explain to me how he had felt trapped, controlled, unhappy and unable to express his feelings. When he caused himself pain in this way, he was in control, he could feel pain in his body, it made sense somehow. It was a physical representation of a pain he could not explain and a pain that he was ashamed of feeling. Other young people explain it as a feeling of something when everything else feels numb. It is often not a precursor to suicide.

Our relationship to our body is fragile in the world of yoga. I believe that social media helps to perpetuate the 'body perfect' myth, which damages so many young people. We are bombarded by edited images of doll-like women pouting in tight lycra, contorting themselves into impossible postures, calling it yoga. This has a dual effect of making it attractive to young people because they want to look like these impossible images and also of actually attracting them to a science that can take them way beyond this surface image, if they are lucky enough to have a teacher who is curious and earnest in their search for the heart of yoga.

Ayurveda

Ayurveda is a complex and broad science of life, which often takes a lifetime to comprehend. It involves all kinds of self-care modalities, including massage, food as medicine, herbal medicine, breathwork, all yoga techniques and much, much more. It is a science that dates back around 5000 years, much like yoga today, and is practised widely in the UK and most countries across the world. It has seen a renaissance in India in the last few years, supported by government initiatives that understand its influence on the world and importance to modern medicine.

In Ayurveda the shape of our body gives the ayurvedic practitioner clues to their character and personality, what they may be able to engage in and how their energy levels are likely to fluctuate, and also which foods they might benefit from and which would be harmful. All these elements differ from individual to individual.

Ayurveda and body types

In Ayurveda there are three body types (or *doshas*), which have always helped me understand my students better: *kapha*, *pitta* and *vata*. Most people are a mixture of these types, and this helps us understand what kind of practice they might benefit from the most. *Kapha* types are naturally heavy set, with large eyes, a comfortable way about them and an open face. *Pitta* types are fiery, critical and active; they are good at getting things done. They are prone to skin conditions and have reddish faces and a mane of hair. *Vata* types are airy and have a tendency to be forgetful and flighty but can have very quick and interesting minds. They tend to have a wiry frame and narrow faces. We are all a combination of these types with more or less of each *dosha*.

***Vata* asana exercises**

Most *vata* types would like to beef up a bit, and they need to stay stable and strong. So the top five asanas for a *vata* type could be:

1. arm balances
2. slow sun salutation
3. warrior held for two minutes
4. *chaturanga*[3]
5. forward bends (to help digestion, ground the body and eliminate *vata*)

***Pitta* asana exercises**

Ideally *pitta* types should do their yoga in the early morning or evening to avoid overheating in the summer. They have a tendency to get hot and bothered, so cooling practices are best, such as:

---

3 *Chaturanga* is a Sanskrit term for a posture sometimes called the 'plank' in English, where the toes and hands support the body which is parallel to the floor.

1. pigeon
2. camel
3. cobra
4. bow
5. fish

Kapha asana exercises

More often than not, a *kapha* person might be a bit too lazy to do asana and feel a bit fed up of being a little overweight, so need it the most. The wonderful thing about *kaphas* is they are so stable and comforting to the rest of us and they are meant to be a little rounder than others. So *kapha* students should try to do an invigorating asana practice to get the energy moving in the body and balance their energies a bit more.

Kapha types should do the practice in the early morning. The practice should include:

1. a quick and mindful sun salutation
2. strong *vinyasa* flow, maybe *ashtanga* or *anusara*[4]
3. half spinal twists to help digestion
4. mostly standing postures, such as dancer
5. bellows breath

General practices for loving your body

Be aware that many students struggling with anorexia nervosa are likely to be looking to lose calories from their practice. In some cases this can be lethal, so try to slow down their practice and make it soothing and self-loving, rather than tough.

---

4 *Ashtanga* yoga is a form of postural yoga which is quite dynamic, involving jumps and advanced flexibility exercises.
Anusara yoga is a form of yoga founded by John Friend who synthesised the *Iyengar* and the *Ashtanga* methods.

Example for class exercises

- Very gentle breathing while lying on their stomachs, feeling breath enter and leave the body.
- Sit up and teach *dirga* breath – or you can call it the ladder breath – where you breathe in one level, hold the breath, breathe in the next level and, finally, the final step of the ladder until your lungs are full. At this point you hold at the top of your breath and let the breath go slowly, like a thread coming out of your mouth – this will help lower anxiety.
- Now coming into cat cow, you move the spine gently, allowing for release along the entire back – this will help the nervous system.
- Coming into downward dog, releasing hamstrings, neck, shoulders and head.
- A slow sun salutation, holding each posture and feeling into the release.
- Coming onto their backs, legs into the belly to release any digestive issues, such as trapped wind, and encouraging healthy digestion. Roll from side to side.
- Sitting up cross legged, do some side stretches to release anger and twists to help digestion again.
- Butterfly, to release emotions, and cradling each leg, to enhance self-compassion.
- Self-massage, hands and arms, feet (if they want to) and legs; lie down on stomach for relaxation.
- Final affirmation:

  May all beings be well.
  May all beings be free from suffering.
  May all beings meet challenges with courage.

— Chapter 9 —

FOOD

For your journal

What is your relationship to food?

Do you ever eat when you are not hungry?

Do you ever punish yourself through withholding food?

Have you ever noticed your health change with your diet?

My battle with bulimia began when I was about 14–15 years old, in Year 10 at school. Surrounded my girls who were all doing various things to keep slim (laxatives, not eating, puking) I was soon to fall into a pattern of overeating and making myself sick. This pattern increased as I reached my 20s and had a baby young. I found it was actually a way to relieve stress. It was around 2003 that I really found yoga. I first found this at the gym I attended and then went on courses and retreats. Soon I was able to develop my own home practice. Although none of this was specifically aiming at overcoming an eating disorder, I did find that through yoga and meditation I was able to cope with stresses more easily and was actually less stressed. I was finding a new love for myself and my body. I just didn't even think to make myself sick any more. I was and am loving my life and body, and I know without yoga I would have not been able to find this as I had been battling the self-loathing and addiction to bulimia for years.

Relationship with food

Our connection with food is emotional because we perceive it to be the most concrete form of nourishment. We perceive it to be the most readily form of *prana* (life force). It also has the role of grounding us. When we eat we can come out of our wandering minds and into our body, which is the conduit to the present moment. Our bodies are present; they host the senses which bring us into awareness of everything around us, the present moment. Our first comfort after leaving the cosy connection with mother is with breast milk and so it continues. We continue to comfort ourselves in times of isolation and loneliness with food. The connection we can experience to food is perhaps the connection with Nature herself, with the life force within any growing plant, fruit or animal. When we consume food we are literally consuming life force to add to our own. What many realise with years of sincere yoga practice is, in fact, that *prana* can be accessible in so many other ways as well; for example, in the breath, in water and in releasing tension in the body, we become aware of released streams of *prana*, like when you unblock a river, it flows abundantly through our being again.

Vegetarianism

Freshly picked fruit and vegetables are full of *prana*. Anything that has been freshly picked and delivered to your plate retains *prana*.

There are several reasons why many yogis choose to become vegetarians or vegans. Many yogis choose a vegetarian or vegan diet as a natural follow-on to their compassion for all living matter. When we start to become aware of our connection with Nature, we no longer want to be responsible for the death of another being. Within the lineages that propound vegetarianism, the main line of argument is fourfold:

1. We don't want to be responsible for the death of other living beings.
2. Our digestion is better suited to a non-meat diet.
3. It is the ecological/ethical/sustainable choice.
4. There is more *prana* in the food.

When our awareness expands to understand our responsibility and connection with all living matter, we no longer want to be responsible for the death of another living being. Eating meat can then feel unnecessarily violent. Meat takes 72 hours to digest whereas vegetables take 12 hours or less. This has an impact on our digestive tract, where food will be putrefying for longer, causing undesirable effects on the lining of the entire tract. It is more sustainable to grow vegetables than to produce meat, in terms of water and space needed. This means that the planet can sustain a vegetarian diet more easily than an animal one. A piece of dead meat has very little *prana*, as the *prana* leaves the body when the animal is killed. It is true to say that fruit and vegetables that have been in the fridge for a while tend to lose *prana* too, but it is possible to get hold of fresh, newly picked vegetables and fruit, bursting with *prana*. Or, even better, grow your own!

Clean eating

In the last few years we have seen a rise in the concept of clean eating – often meaning coming close to the original and optimal state of food, as it comes out of the ground. It seems clear to me that this is a reaction against an increasingly processed food culture. Some of us simply yearn to return to basics and eat what we can trust to be good, pure food.

However, it does tend to feed into a diet-driven class system, which heralds the slim as somehow purer, 'cleaner', which makes the rest of us 'dirty'! The clear judgement in this manipulative language is dangerously under the radar for many of us and needs to be exposed. We need to have a certain epistemic vigilance, noticing the impact on our minds when using the word 'clean'.

Young people and food

I have found many of my young yogis to be particularly curious and a little confused about what to eat. They have been brought up in a school system that has accentuated healthy eating, yet they are bombarded with sugary, processed foods. To keep things simple and allow for a relaxed attitude around food, I simply say – as much fresh food as possible! Due to their propensity to eat processed, salty and sugary foods, many teens suffer quite badly from constipation. In fact, I was shocked to hear from one of my students, who is a paediatrician in an accident and emergency department, that the most common reason teens come in to hospital is severe constipation. They present with a host of seemingly unrelated issues – stomach cramping, gas, severe headaches, backache, inability to think straight, lethargy but inability to sleep. So below I have sequenced some asana to help with digestion.

Subtle aspects of food

In yoga ashrama we always chant while cooking and also before eating. The reason for this is to acknowledge that the intention while cooking and eating will impact how we integrate the goodness into our bodies and our souls. If the food has been cooked with love and with the intention of nourishing and nurturing us, then this intention is more important than the actual food itself. We see beyond what is on the plate to the heart of the person who created it. When you start to see food in this way, you will take a much closer look at the chef!

Self-respect and yoga

The main benefit of yoga practice in relation to food is that, if done correctly, we can regulate our relationship with food, seeking comfort and discipline in postures, balancing the breath and deep relaxation, which brings about a deep sense of relief. The act of coming to yoga is an act of self-respect and a return to the balance of ease and wellbeing. Therefore, our relationship to food becomes less emotional and more pragmatic.

Exercise for helping with the practice of eating mindfully

When you eat, take your time and focus on the practice of eating mindfully. This entails:

1. Choosing your food carefully, choosing fresh-looking produce that is ready to eat.

2. Preferably buying food from local and organic producers.
3. Minimising foods that have travelled from faraway countries.
4. Preparing food thoughtfully – try to always eat with someone else, so that there is an aspect of offering (sometimes at home, we take some out to the homeless shelter in our town).
5. Eating with reverence, aware of the journey the food has taken to get to your table.
6. Eating in silence, savouring each morsel, by first looking at it, smelling it, tasting it and then swallowing it. Many yogis prefer to eat with their hands, as then you get to feel your food as well. The *prana* of your hands will also come into the food and lend it more love and life force.
7. Taking some time to digest. Preferably you need 20 minutes to digest your food in silence or while taking a slow walk, to help the blood flow in the body and avoid lethargy later on in the day.
8. Checking your bowel movements: you should ideally be going to the toilet before each meal easily and smoothly.
9. Aiding digestion: you could drink hot water before the meal.

Asana and breathing for digestion

Breathing exercise

Bhastrika – pumping the diaphragm for a few minutes. This is done by audibly and forcefully sucking in the air in through the nostrils with some force and then exhaling with similar force, as if you are blowing your nose. The belly should be moving; if only the chest is moving, then you need to start again with abdominal breathing. Out on the inhalation and in during the exhalation. The student needs to be completely comfortable with belly breathing before doing this exercise. This is known as a *kriya* – a cleansing technique. It moves the bowel and wakes up the mind (the two are very much linked).

This *kriya* can be done initially for just a few breaths. If the student feels dizzy or uncomfortable, then they need to stop immediately. As they get used to it, it is a good *kriya* to do every morning before breakfast for a minute or two.

Contra-indication: Do not use this breath with anyone who has panic attacks or severe anxiety.

Asana exercise

- Lying down on the back, hug the knees into the chest and roll from side to side.
- Supine, with the back flat on the floor, move the bent legs from side to side, like a windscreen wiper. (This can be done for several minutes.)
- On all fours, cat cow, tucking belly in for the exhalation and letting it drop towards the floor for the inhalation.
- Seated twist, one leg out in front of you and the other bent with knee up towards the ceiling and foot by the knee. Twist the body towards the bent knee as far as you can go, placing the leading hand on the floor, while the trailing hand squeezes the knee into the abdomen. Hold this posture for a minute or so.
- Do this on the other side.
- Come to squatting, knees to the side, elbows pressing onto the inside of the knees and palms together.
- Roll onto the stomach and grab the feet behind you for the bow; roll from side to side.
- Push up into child's pose.
- Rest here.

— Chapter 10 —

ANXIETY

For your journal

Have you ever felt anxious?

Where in your body have you felt it?

How do you calm yourself?

I'd flunked my first year and had to repeat at another school. Most of my friends had dropped out completely and were doing apprenticeships, but my parents believed in me, and the school agreed, after a lot of resistance, to give me a second chance. But as I approached the school on the first day in September, my heart pounded, my hands went clammy. I had to stop outside, everyone was just walking past. I pretended I was OK, but I couldn't speak, I couldn't move, I couldn't do anything. It was like I was paralysed, on the spot. All I could feel was my heart like it was about to jump out of my chest. I turned around and went straight home. The next day I managed to overcome the anxiety and walk into the school. My mum's friend had taught me to just focus on my breath, look at one spot on the wall, like, just stare at it, so everything else goes away. It worked. (Neall, 17)

Definition of anxiety

Anxiety is defined as a feeling of worry, nervousness or unease about something with an uncertain outcome. It is a widespread problem among adults and, in the last decade or so, has filtered down to affect children and adolescents to a very large degree, affecting about 1 in 3 14–17-year-olds. Women are twice as likely to have anxiety than men, according to statistics offered by the Mental Health Foundation.[1] It is by far the most common issue that yoga therapists and teachers are faced with. The physiological factors (chronic activation of the sympathetic nervous system) resulting from anxiety and stress can cause severe illness and dis-ease (not being at ease) in the body and mind, such as IBS, high blood pressure, heart attacks and most inflammatory diseases. Have you ever thought about how we combat anxiety in the West? We will often reach for the chocolate bar or the biscuit tin. We might phone a friend or text someone. We might binge watch a favourite series or drink alcohol or take drugs. What do you do when you are feeling anxious?

Anxiety is a physiological experience, we can sense it in our body, it causes stress – the heart races, our hands get clammy, we project into the future about all the horrendous things that may or may not happen to us or a loved one. We are projecting into the future with apprehension and worry. Often, many of these worries are completely ungrounded. Anxiety can be caused by a traumatic event which we may or may not remember. It can be a way of seeing the world as a dangerous place, full of unexpected fearful events.

Causes of anxiety

Some young people are anxious due to the kind of food they are or are not eating – food has an impact on mood as most of our hormones are secreted in the gut (vitamins B6 and B12 as well as magnesium have a massive impact on mood). It can also be due to recreational drug use, which impacts their mental state. Many are ungrounded in their bodies, disconnected from themselves. Some are harbouring trauma which causes them anxiety, and some have inherited an anxiety habit, passed down from generation to generation.

Do you remember the eight limbs of yoga from earlier? These eight essential steps of the ladder that lead us to calm and optimal wellness could be inverted to understand how we come to anxiety, which is the opposite to optimal wellness.

---

1 Martin-Merino *et al.* 2009.

It is an interesting exercise to invert the eight limbs to find out what might make us the opposite of blissed (opposite of *samadhi*) – I guess the list might look a bit like this:

1. no ethical codes in relation to my society
2. no moral codes to guide myself
3. no physical practice or discipline
4. no awareness of breath
5. no reflection or introspection, complete reliance on the senses
6. lack of focus
7. a scattered mind
8. anxiety.

Not all of the causes are present in anxiety, but often you will find some of the above elements are present in someone who has anxiety.

This is a good exercise to do with young people: get them to draw up a flowchart of how to become anxious and then one on how to become well, being sure to define wellness as closely as possible. Which steps do we need to take in order to be well, to feel 'zen'?

One of the most common reasons students find their way to yoga is because of anxiety. If caught early on, yoga exercises can prove to be a supportive practice that may well stave off any more dramatic expressions of anxiety later on in life and help control this debilitating and all too common state. If we fail to curb anxiety, it can lead to not coping in general with life or, specifically, when we are teenagers, it has an impact on sleep, exams, academic performance and friendships, and our physical and mental health in general will be deeply affected.

> Young people experience a great deal of pressure, and consequently stress, to perform well in school due to the high expectations on them both academically and socially. Yoga is a great way to deal with this and the Teen Yoga Programme has been extremely well received by students at Ralph Allen. The approach taken is just

right and has inspired our students not just to try yoga, but to stick with it. I recommend the programme wholeheartedly. (John Chantry, Vice Principal, Ralph Allen School, Bath)

Many yoga teachers and therapists are of the opinion that a good relaxation will support an anxious person. However, in my experience, anxiety requires a strong practice first. And not just any kind of strong practice but a practice that targets specific muscles in specific ways and order.

Preparation exercise for the therapist

A practice for you for protection and courage – do a short grounding meditation and asana practice before the students enter. Grounding is essential for the yoga teacher and therapist before this class or session. Maybe you have a mantra you could use, or you could simply repeat, during your exercises, *grounded and strong, grounded and strong.*

Class exercises

Some of these practices are harder than others, some more suited to more active people, others to quieter people; pick what's best for your student.

Step one

The first step for anxious students is to put them at ease by listening to their story.

Step two

The next step is not getting into the story!

Step three

Now for some vigorous exercises, depending on their ability.

Anxiety is fight or flight, it is the body getting vigilant because of a perceived threat. Therefore certain muscles are activated by the cortisol which floods the bloodstream. Mostly we notice that the large muscles in the thighs and the upper arms become tense and ready for conflict or escape.

- So we need to activate these muscles effectively – starting in chair pose, with the arms elevated, allows for these muscles to be activated.
- Then move slowly through the sun salutation, accentuating any postures using these two muscle groups.
- Coming to the end, use some static poses to again accentuate these groups, such as plank and chair or high lunge.
- Use the *ujjayi* breath,[2] which has three benefits:

  Lengthening the outbreath will start to calm the nervous system.

  It also invigorates the mind and body.

  It brings the student into *pratyahara*, an inward-looking state.
- Make sure the heart rate is raised and there is a sense of working hard – this is important for the anxiety to release.
- When you notice that the student is puffing a bit, then you can start the static postures, burning off the last cortisol in the muscle groups.
- At this stage you can start to focus more on the outbreath, as they come down into child's pose (for safety and security) – ask them if they need a blanket over their back. Many young people find *savasana* too vulnerable in the beginning, so child's pose is a great option. Also, in child's pose we are encouraging inward focus and awareness of breath in the back of the body.
- Come up to sitting or kneeling and roll the shoulders and stretch the neck – we all hold a whole lot of tension here

---

2 *Ujjayi* breath is also known as Darth Vader breath, where you half close the back of the throat and breathe in and out with some force. There is a little friction in the back of the throat while breathing.

when we are anxious. End with the eye roll. Take some time over this and keep the head still.

- Now, focusing on the back, do the cat cow on all fours or sitting up, as you are on the knees, if that feels more appropriate for a beginner.
- Gauge how much time you do this, from around two minutes to five.
- Standing up slowly, come into a standing forward fold. Accentuate the outbreath, the letting go; you can use a useful narrative of letting thoughts drop out of your head and into the floor, letting go of the lower spine. Again, lengthening the outbreath.
- When this has been done, if there is still some anxiety, you can repeat a few lunges and then come down to lying on the floor to increase grounding, then do a supine twist, releasing any residual tension in the spine. Allow legs to bend at the knee and drop alternately left and right, very slowly, keeping the legs in this position for five breaths each. Make sure the back is flat on the floor. Press gently with the opposite hand on the opposite knee.
- By this stage they may be ready for a relaxation – check in with them, not verbally, but listen to their breathing and look at their face; you should be able to tell if they are at a state ready to relax.
- If they are comfortable and feel safe, go ahead and ask them to lie on their back, but otherwise lie on their tummy. Guide them back to their breath, slowly and steadily.
- Explain exactly what is going to happen next, that they will be lying still and you will be scanning the body and asking them to mentally relax all the limbs in turn and that it will take between two and five minutes, after which they might feel a bit spaced out.
- Now body scan – from the feet to the crown, take a good ten minutes, if they are relaxed, to relax the whole body. If they still seem a little agitated it is important to do this

relatively quickly so it doesn't become something they do not like.

- Use blankets, bolsters, eye pillows or anything that might make them more comfortable.
- When they come out of the relaxation, which will need to be done very gently, please do not engage in discussion but, when they are in the liminal state, you can encourage them to be aware of their state and how it is to feel calm and relaxed and that that is a normal state which they can reach at any given moment.
- Try not to chat too much at the end of class but allow them to leave quietly, when they are ready. If you are doing this in a school, be sure that they are fully awake before the bell sounds. If they have class after, make them roll onto their left side; if they are going home get them to lie on their right side. Let them understand the value of silence and stillness.

Don't assume they have had the experience you want them to have – they may have found it unpleasant or difficult; give them space for that too.

When your students have had a few positive experiences and are managing to go deeper into the *savasana*, then prolong the *savasana*. Initially it might be as short as 2–3 minutes; don't worry if they giggle or fidget, it is just them getting used to the exercise.

When they are comfortable in *savasana* and able to go deep, then go on to the next steps.

Step four

Out of my mind – yoga *nidra*

Here is a script that I wrote for young people (if there are boys in the class, you can change the word woman to person):

Garden of blossom

Welcome home

Lay flat, feeling the earth beneath you, like the roots of interlaced flowers that you spread out, reaching down into the earth, that belongs to you and your body

Close the eyes

Exhale and allow the body to settle

Feel the breath becoming spacious, slow and steady

Allow the body to be breathed by the trees and the air around you, pulsating in unison with all life

As you breathe out, the trees breathe in; as the tree breathes out you breathe in, belonging to nature

Settling the body into effortless stillness, deep stillness

Be aware: 'I am practising yoga *nidra*, I am practising yoga *nidra*, I am practising yoga *nidra*'

Repeat your intention or you can use this one:

'I am grounded and connected, I am grounded and connected, I am grounded and connected'

Let this be a form of awareness

Be held by this state of consciousness

Be safe within the vessel of the form of awareness which is yoga *nidra*

Exhale – drop the mind down into the heart

Let the awareness be deep in the heart

'I am my heart, I am my heart, I am my own true heart, my heart is wide open'

Welcome the feelings and insights that arise in the heart

Welcome the voice of the inner teacher

Guide now the light of conscious awareness around the body

The body remains still but the awareness moves from point to point

It is as if the body belongs to the ground

The light of mental attention shines at each point

Awakening the bright presence of a new growth in the ground

So the body becomes a web of interlaced flowers and opening blooms

Inhale, the breath moves out to all the flowers

Let a flower blossom at each point

At the crown of the head

Between the eyebrows, in the throat, between the collarbones

Shine the bright light of awareness down the right arm and watch how the blooms open along the arm

Shoulder, elbow, wrist, thumb, index finger, middle finger, ring finger, little finger and back

Inside the right wrist, elbow, shoulder

Bring the awareness back to the throat, between the collarbones

Shine the bright light of awareness down the left arm

Shoulder, elbow, wrist, thumb, index finger, middle finger, ring finger, little finger and back

Inside the left wrist, elbow, shoulder

Bring the awareness back to the throat, between the collarbones

Shine the awareness down into the heart space

A bright full flower in the middle of the chest, behind the breastbone, a deep red rose

Drop the awareness down to the navel, let the awareness shine there and watch a blossom bloom

Drop the awareness to your pelvis, let the awareness shine there, watch the flower bloom

Shine the awareness over the right hip, and feel a trail of flowers opening down the right leg

Knee, ankle, big toe, second toe, third toe, fourth toe, little toe

And back inside, flowers blooming in the right ankle, knee and hip

Bring the awareness back to the blossom in the pelvis

Shine the awareness over the left hip, and feel a trail of flowers opening down the left leg

Knee, ankle, big toe, second toe, third toe, fourth toe, little toe

And back inside, flowers blossoming in the left ankle, knee and hip

Bring the awareness back to the blossom in the pelvis

Bring the awareness back to the navel and the bright light, allowing the flower to blossom there

Bring the awareness back to the deep heart and the flower there

Be clear: 'I am practising yoga *nidra*, I am practising yoga *nidra*, I am practising yoga *nidra*'

Be aware of the whole body and the garden of flowers growing and blossoming in every space, a garden of blossoms, the whole body

Inhale, the space between the flowers open

So more flowers fill the space

Exhale, the petals fall to the earth, settling in a pattern on the body

Inhale, flowers rise and spread, spacious open dark between them

Exhale, light allows the petals to drop like light rain

Landing on the garden of the body, resting on the earth

Light dawns

Feel the petal drops warmed on the body as the sun shines

Inhale, the earth is warmed

The petals on the body, released by the fire in the sky

Exhale, petals fall to the earth

Inhale, flowers reach for the sky

Exhale into the roots

Pause between the breaths

With awareness in the magnificent rose at the centre of the heart space

Awareness in the anchor roots, heels, hands

Awareness in the anchor roots – legs and arms

Awareness in the spine and the head

Breathing on the web of roots, anchored in the earth, breathing flowers into being

Let the bright light of consciousness travel triangles in the body web of roots

Exhale, breath moves down from the pelvis to the heels

Inhale, breath moves up from heels to pelvis

Upward-pointing triangle

Pause to exhale, awareness at the pelvis

Inhale, breath moves up from pelvis to chest

Exhale, breath moves down from chest to pelvis

Inhale, breath returns to chest

Pause to exhale, awareness at chest

Downward-pointing triangle

Inhale, breath moves up from chest to eyebrow centre, like a rhizome finding its way

Exhale, breath moves down from eyebrow centre to chest

Inhale, breath moves up to eyebrow centre

Upward-pointing triangle

Let conscious awareness join the upward-pointing triangle

To the downward-pointing triangle

They meet at the chest

Let the breath move in the diamond of the body root web

Blossoming diamond of flowers

Exhale from the eyebrow centre to the chest

And pause to inhale

Exhale from the chest to the pelvis

Inhale from the pelvis to the chest

And pause to exhale

Inhale from the chest to eyebrow centre

Exhale back to chest

Breath awareness consciousness in the diamond

Diamond breath makes the shape vivid

A bright diamond of awareness

'I am practising yoga *nidra*, I am practising yoga *nidra*, I am practising yoga *nidra*'

Then

Exhale all awareness, from the edges of the diamond into the heart space

In the centre of the diamond

Inhale awareness outward to the edges of the diamond of flowers

And back to the full rose of the heart space

Being in the heart space in the diamond, in the web

Feeling the flowers blossoming

'I am my heart, I am my heart, I am my own true heart, and my heart is open!'

Breathe awareness into the heart space

Welcome the insights of the inner teacher, carried on the silent voice of the inner teacher

Welcome home to yourself

Repeating your intention again:

'I am grounded and connected, I am grounded and connected, I am grounded and connected'

Woman on the web of dreams

Integrated

Laying like a web of flowers

Safe in the consciousness that is yoga *nidra*

Securely held by this experience

Safe within the vessel of the form of awareness which is yoga *nidra*

Know that this practice of yoga *nidra* is coming to an end

Carry the blessings of the practice, the awareness of connection out with you

The practice of yoga *nidra* is complete

Stretch, yawn and open your eyes

Let your breath be a bridge to a more everyday state of consciousness

Yet savour still the bright presence of awareness

Hari Om Tat Sat

Step five

WITNESSING

Teach them to watch their thoughts, be the witness with utter compassion, noticing anger if it is there (or any other so-called positive or negative emotion), maybe see if it belongs anywhere in the body, whether it has a shape, a colour, a pulsation; notice it, breathe into it and have respect and love for it as it were their own child. Notice the space between emotions and thoughts. Notice their breathing as you do this.

Time: 5–20 minutes

Step six

SING YOUR HEART OUT

Chanting om or other chants (lengthens the outbreath and is a wonderful way to express emotions); with om you can simply start as a humming breath – or the Brahmari breath and move on from there – expressing sound is very therapeutic, and expressing it together with someone can be wonderfully uplifting, especially if there is no pressure on it sounding great.

You could sing along with Krishna Das, MC Yogi or similar.

Step seven

CHANGING YOUR MIND

This is a lovely Buddhist exercise, which helps us work on the idea that we can change our thoughts and also helps us exercise compassion towards ourselves and others.

Metta:[3]

- Think of someone you love (not a boyfriend or girlfriend) and send them kindness, imagine smiling at them in the place you normally see them, maybe even giving them a hug.

---

3 *Metta* means loving kindness or benevolence in Pali, the language of Buddha, and is one of the main practices in mindfulness exercises.

- Repeat: 'May you be well and happy, may you overcome challenges with ease.'
- Now move onto someone you like and do the same thing.
- Next, someone who you don't feel specially anything for and do the same thing.
- Then move onto a relative and repeat.
- Then move onto someone you don't know very well at all and repeat.
- Then imagine someone you don't like very much and imagine smiling warmly at them, sincerely.
- Finally, imagine meeting yourself and doing this too.
- Notice if any of these were tricky and be kind to yourself.

Time: 10 minutes

Step eight

SLOWING DOWN (*DIRGA* BREATH)

Breathe in deeply in three parts, first part to the navel, second part to the chest and third part to the clavicles, and then breathe out super slowly making a sound like the ocean (*ujjayi* breath).

Time: 10 minutes

Step nine

CHILLING OUT

Breathe in for six seconds and out for six seconds for 20 minutes (make a timer on your phone, like a gentle mindfulness bell sound). Notice the stillness that descends on you.

Time: 20 minutes

Suggestions for home exercises

Taking care

Self-massage (*abyangha*) with warm oils such as sesame oil or almond oil (add some rosemary if you need cheering up or lavender for deeper relaxing) or massaging with a friend. (If with a friend you can stick to the back, legs, arms and hands and feet; if by yourself, you include the whole body.) Or would they let you massage them? Then lie with your legs up the wall for five minutes, while listening to your favourite music.

Time: 10–30 minutes

Having fun

A few of your favourite postures, from one of the online resources, such as the TeenYoga YouTube channel, Charlottayogi or Yoga Glo, or YouTube generally, followed by a thorough body scan and *savasana*. Try some partner postures too with your friend or a family member.

Time: 10–20 minutes

Yoga *nidra*

— Chapter 11 —

DEPRESSION

For your journal

How do you recognise depression in someone?

What are the factors that lead to a depressive episode, in your experience?

How can yoga support someone with depression?

How do you take care of yourself when working with someone who has depression?

I had always been the top of my class, I played as a soloist in the school orchestra, I was popular and got the highest marks. I was on the A team for hockey. Then I got into the top university, and suddenly I was no one. Everyone else seemed so much more confident than me, they had more friends than me, I didn't fit in. Everyone played an instrument to a higher standard than me and played sports on the university team. My grades plummeted, I painted my room black, I started missing lectures, I started drinking. I partied myself to destruction. One day I found myself in prison. I had been caught driving my sister and her friend to the shopping centre, so drunk that I can't even remember doing it. They were 14. I could have killed them. My parents were beside themselves with worry. I was sent to prison. There was yoga there. Slowly I started to feel alive again. This woman came every week and was so kind and compassionate. I started to feel my body, became aware of my breath. I felt like a flower blossoming, a flower that had been underground for so many years, now exposed to the sun for

> the first time. I wanted to be like her, I wanted to be light, kind and good. I started doing yoga in my room. I became stronger and stronger. And here I am today, a yoga instructor. When you have learned a skill like yoga, you have to share it with others; if it can make people better, like it did me, you have to. (RT, 19 years old)

Definition of depression

Defined as a feeling of severe dejection and despondency, depression among young people is on the rise. The number of teens each year who have a depressive episode went up by 37 per cent between 2005 and 2014.[1] Depression and anxiety are often mentioned in the same breath, because long-term anxiety can be a precursor to depression. In depression, we are often lingering on past events, looking backwards with regret, grief or sorrow, while in anxiety we are looking forward in trepidation. Once we have come into a depressive state, typified by low serotonin, GABA and dopamine levels in the brain, it is difficult to rise again. Fear, listlessness and apathy become our bedfellows, and nothing matters, not even getting better. For depressed teens, yoga could be the answer. When nothing helps, and nothing matters, moving the body can feel good and could definitely be the first step towards seeing a little light at the end of the tunnel. The principles here are very different from the anxious state. The *rajas* of anxiety has been king for too long and exhausted the system into *tamas*. In biological terms, the chronic stress of anxiety has resulted in a fatigued system, which no longer has the energy to be inflamed, heightened and alert.

> I feel we have all become softer, happier, and it has made a difference to the staff too; they have more tolerance towards each other, they can listen to each other better. (Teacher)

Common causes of depression

Clinical depression is a debilitating disease, brought on by a variety of factors, including trauma, circumstance and nutrition. It is commonly characterised by low self-esteem, loss of interest, low

---

1 Mojtabai, Olfson and Han 2016.

energy as well as physical and mental pain – it impacts every area of life. There is no magic pill; the factors that precede a depressive episode are often numerous, diverse and particularly personal. From a yoga perspective, we recognise it as an extreme form of *tamas*. I worked for a while exclusively with sectioned service users at the Callington Road Hospital in Bristol, those who had been sectioned because they were either harming themselves or someone else. Most of them were diagnosed with severe depression. This was heavy work and not something I would recommend anyone to take on lightly. The over-riding common thread that I noticed among these students of yoga was abuse of drugs and/or addiction. In most cases I believe that this was brought about by the trauma that they had experienced, usually during their younger years. By trauma we normally mean psychological trauma, brought about by emotional or sexual abuse or neglect.

Physical aspects of depression

The physical aspects of depression tend to be lethargy, lack of desire to move or be active, chronic pain (often in the back) but also somatisation (feeling a specific pain, localised to a specific area, but no medical explanation), together with a lack of desire to open up the body. Depressed young people should be an oxymoron – this time of exploration, new friendships, new learning and new environments, all seem anathema to the *tamas*ic experience of depression. Sadly, they are not, often because in young people there is such a long-term overload of anxiety, which can lead to depression. I also believe that sometimes the overidentification with the body and the senses, therefore the reliance on outside stimuli to give information, leads many along a path towards comparison, negativity about body image and so on. In turn this exacerbates the mind's propensity to compare, contrast, ruminate, all of which are highly problematic. When the mind turns inwards to itself, guided and nurtured on the way by an expert teacher who sees us with an unconditional positive regard, we can integrate experiences, emotions and thought and eventually come to a place of silence, beauty and stillness. The more we practise coming towards this inward fluid and reflective state with compassion, the less likely we are to be influenced by outward stimuli and others' opinions and subsequent ruminations and mind wandering.

As with all states, we meet the students where they are, so, if they are feeling low, it is important to meet them at that state and take them gently to another experience, as far as they are willing.

Our job as therapists is to gently wake the system up again, feeling into sensations and feelings as they arise, without judgement or the desire to 'fix' them, guiding them into a calm and compassionate state. Using the step-ladder approach, we would ideally be addressing fundamental values as stipulated in the *yamas* and *niyamas*, during our asana class.

Class exercises

1. Avoid asking how they are feeling – this can be a stressful question. Most of your communication will be intuitive and non-verbal. Make them very welcome. Make sure they feel completely safe in the room by indicating where they can sit, but give them a choice. Sit them where they can see the door, where they know what is around them; you might like to explain where the toilet is, and any fire exits and so on. Ask if they want a drink of water.

2. If they feel comfortable, bring them to the mat on their stomach or in child's pose.

3. From here, they can start to rock the body, side to side.

   (In forward bends we are creating and accentuating safety, with the rocking we are creating comfort.)

4. Be very cautious with any opening postures or any strengthening postures as they are likely to feel weak and protective.

5. Bring attention to the breath while on the stomach – this is a good place to practise breathing, as you can feel it in the back and in the sides of the body. The breath is always with us, our constant companion, rhythmical and kind. We can change the breath and change our mood; teach them this first of all. So deepen the breath which is likely to be shallow

and uneven, and lengthen the outbreath. Tears are plentiful when we struggle with depression, they come often and copiously – let them come. Try not to comfort or mention them, it often makes the client feel uncomfortable. Maybe just a hand on their back, if that feels right.

6. Next, start to stretch the body in the forward fold, so lengthen the back and the arms reaching out in front and then one side and the other.
7. Lengthen the legs out underneath the body, into a forward bend. You might be surprised at how stiff young people can be in the forward bend, in which case, offer a block for them to sit on and a strap to connect with their feet.
8. From here come into crouching, allowing the hips to widen and the body to drop in between the legs and hands on the ground.
9. The element of grounding is beautiful and important in depression, feeling something solid, that is not going to change, that has no quality. Placing hands on the floor and feet on the floor, bring full awareness to the energy flowing through hands and feet into the floor and drawing energy up from the earth into the body, so the reciprocity of energy in all things.
10. Stick the bottom up in the air for a standing forward fold (accentuating again the forward bend and the folding over, which creates safety).
11. Try a warrior at this point; notice how wide the legs are from each other, and this might give you an indication of how strong or grounded they are feeling today. If their legs are far apart then they are feeling strong today – notice and comment on this. Accentuate the awareness of feet on and into the ground.
12. Try a wide-angled forward bend from here, again accentuating the experience of feet and hands on the ground and what's under the floor, the earth, water, mud...
13. Come down to a one-legged forward bend each side.

14. Finish with legs up the wall – a deeply restorative posture – focusing on the breath, maybe with a cushion on the stomach or maybe just the hands. Make the breath as deep as possible.

15. Visualisation might be nice in this posture – visualise relieving the body and the mind of unwanted emotions and thoughts, tuning into the light deep inside the heart. Maybe visualise a bright light at the bottom of your heart, lighting up your entire body cell by cell.

    (With visualisation, it is important to remember that you have no power over what they are actually thinking and one of the more debilitating aspects of depression is the lack of power over thought. Another aspect of depression is the rumination, the mind wandering off to images, memories and imagined situations that make the student feel bad in one way or another. We need to gently coax some kind of discipline to the mind, or even start the idea that we have some kind of control over our thoughts, emotions and therefore behaviour. Visualisation lends this discipline – when practised in a relaxed state, the mind is more able to follow a less vigilant path, a new path towards light and stillness, which is our ultimate goal as practitioners and teachers.)

16. Finish the class off with a lie down, whether on their tummies or on their backs, making sure they feel secure, either with blankets and eye pillows or music and bolsters, whatever is right for the people in front of you.

17. During relaxation, make sure you keep repeating words like the light, and letting go; these two basic terms can really make a difference to the group. Do not pause for too long, as this will let the unwanted thoughts come in again.

I love the idea that when we are depressed, we need deep rest! Deep rest from our thoughts!

If you get a smile, you've done a really good job! If you haven't, you probably have as well.

As with most yoga teaching, getting out of your own way and setting the intention of healing are two of the most important things to remember.

Self-care

If, when you are working with this group, you notice yourself internalising the low mood vibe and taking it with you, make sure you take some time out to do your own practice and maybe sometimes take a break too. I find it helps to take a long walk in nature or a long shower or sauna to cleanse yourself of unwanted emotions and sensations left over from the class.

— Chapter 12 —

ADDICTION

For your journal

Have you ever experienced addiction to a substance?

If so, what purpose does or did that addiction serve?

Have you experienced sharing your life with an addict?

If so, how did it affect you?

Before I started practising, I was a walking collection of addictive behaviours. Drugs and alcohol being the primary culprits. In reflection, I know I was searching for a way to manage my feelings and experiences, but to me, at the time, that just meant numbing them.

I threw myself headfirst into a whirlwind of drinking, drugs and endless, endless parties. It was the ultimate hiding place! The good parts were amazing and the bad...well...I could blame that on the hangover! Eventually fun turned into fear, the parties stopped being interesting, instead I was using in my bedroom, on my own, numb and miserable. As cliché as it sounds, I just wanted an escape.

I guess that's where the dependency started. I left home and dropped out of school, telling myself that 'it wasn't the right path for me'... In reality, it was just getting much too in the way of my using. Eventually, my body couldn't take any more. I woke up in a hospital bed, a drip in my arm, a haze in my head and my stomach aching from the pumping procedure. I'd overdosed and couldn't remember a thing.

> It was after that overdose that I realised I needed to find a way out. This time, I had been lucky, once more and who knew what could happen? The hospital referred me to the youth support centre, The Hive, where I first discovered yoga.
>
> I remember lying on my mat at the end of my first session, my body buzzing with endorphins. Cat, my new-found teacher, was gently coaxing us to close our eyes for *savasana* and let the practice sink in, but I couldn't possibly. I was far too excited. I stared up at the ceiling, elated. This yoga stuff was amazing!
>
> I started practising regularly; I think initially the feeling at the end of the practice was what I was doing it for but, as the weeks progressed, the rush became less important. I started noticing other benefits. I began to feel a sense of myself in the different postures. Warrior was no longer just the name for the pose, it was how I felt when I held it...and that followed me off the mat too. I could be a warrior anywhere. The breathing, the attention and the awareness became my rocks. (LS, 18-year-old woman from London)

Definition of addiction

Addiction is when we are addicted to (i.e. dependent on) a substance or activity, most commonly (according to the US website addiction.com) coffee, gambling, anger, food, the internet, sex, alcohol, drugs, nicotine or work. Addiction is often explained as a chemical dependency; the commonly implicated chemical is dopamine, which is released in copious quantities when we take cocaine or have sex, for example. In my experience I see addiction as a natural follow-on from a life-saving coping mechanism that the individual has found to cope with everyday life and then, like a crutch, they daren't or cannot let go, until they have found an alternative way of coping with the issue that caused them to look for the crutch in the first place. The reasons are multiple, ranging from social shyness and awkwardness to unspecified pain.

It feels important to speak about addiction in the context of young people and yoga, as this is the time of life, with plenty of new experiences, that can lead to the need for coping mechanisms. In turn, these coping mechanisms can lead to addictive habits when repeated. When we feel in pain, or under stress or duress, we repeat what has worked in the past and these habits become part of our character, and naturally, if unquestioned, lead to a lifetime of unhealthy habits.

When and how does addiction start?

Adolescence is a natural time for curiosity and experimentation, with plenty of opportunities to try alcohol, drugs and experiences of different sorts. Why do some children get stuck and others manage to sail through this time and out the other side, unscathed? Is there a profile for the addicted child?

The foundation of addictive behaviour is sometimes laid during the childhood that lacks stability, understanding, guidance and secure attachment. Secure attachment involves a child having constant understanding and feeling seen and heard by a specific carer, preferably the mother. If this is not present in the family, the child will have what is called an insecure or chaotic attachment, which, in turn, can lead to a deep sense of anxiety and loneliness, often experienced as not being understood. When homes are chaotic, they lack stability and lead us to feeling unsure of what is coming next, an outburst of anger, reprimand or anxiety – maybe our primary carer is suddenly not available to take us to school, or has forgotten our packed lunch, or our PE kit. When the parent/carer is chaotic, it becomes frightening to be a child. In a situation like this our adult cannot guide us towards worthwhile goals and protect us from unhelpful actions or habits. Life becomes painful and confusing; the child looks for a way to cope.

Anxiety/emotional intelligence and addiction

The mind is the culprit; when we are constantly ransacked by fear of inadequacy, anxiety about the future or confusion then it becomes impossible to control actions or reactions – the present moment is an impossible place to be. When we are drowned by the inner critic we long for an escape. Sometimes this is framed as an escape from 'reality' – but which reality? What is reality in this context? It is the reality of my own mind chatter. With a little meta-awareness, we can learn to retain a dual focus of attention;

simultaneously aware of my own story as well as being fully aware of the bigger story, where I am only one of many players.

Connection versus addiction

Feeling connected is the true experience of life, connected to the rhythms of nature, the lunar cycle, our circadian rhythms, to the people and animals around us and to the work we do. Also, when our mind is relaxed, we are able to come into the flow and feel acceptance for whatever is happening right now; whether it is 'good' or 'bad', we know it is for the best. Truth flows naturally without fear of judgement. When we are in the flow and our inner critic is side-stepped, we feel connected to others because, just as the criticism levelled at ourselves has subsided, so has the criticism of others – we have come into a space of full acceptance of others. When we are able to do that, we feel connection, love and inclusion into all life. The pain and confusion associated with unreliable adults or carers, or associated with unreliable emotions and reactions, subsides as we come into a witness state of the river of emotions that is constantly flowing. Many yoga therapists see connection as the antidote to addiction for this reason.

Whatever we have 'chosen' to be our addiction has served a purpose – it has helped us to move away from or numb the sense of helplessness, loneliness or unworthiness.

Addiction to what?

It is common to think of addiction in terms of alcohol, drugs, social media, sexual behaviour, destructive relationships or gambling, the areas which have had a lot of focus over the past 50 years or so, but the subtler and more socially acceptable or invisible addictions may be the more insidious, such as addiction to sugar, work, screen time or pornography, which have just as deleterious effects on relationships as the more obvious addictive substances. Young people today have access to many varied substances, ranging from cannabis (which around 86% of 14-year-olds in the UK have tried) to ketamine and other as yet untested drugs.[1] These are all of

---

1 Macleod *et al.* 2004.

great concern, as any habit that we embed in our daily or weekly rhythm at this age has a very high certainty of staying with us into adulthood. But, if we take it to a subtler level, we can see that we are 'addicted' to certain thought patterns that will have a long-term effect on both character and destiny. The underlying factor, which we may call fear of isolation, is where our focus needs to be, rather than which substance is used to mitigate and dull the experience.

> *Mainly I have noticed that I am calmer, more relaxed and much more careful [due to yoga] and I transmit that to my friends and those around me.* (Carlos, 15)

Social media

This is a new one for many of us, only really coming to the fore in the last ten years or so when mobile phones and tablets have flooded the lives of our young people. It is hard to get a perspective on the importance and impact of social media on us and them at this stage. It is here to stay – I see many adults who seem to be more addicted than the younger generation, who have developed necessary strategies of ignoring the constant messaging and notifications coming through. In my experience I have found that the more studious and focused students, who have lots of support from home and school, tend to have a higher resistance to the draw of social media, whereas those with low levels of attention, who are often disengaged and disinterested in school, will be easily distracted by the little jolts of notifications throughout the day and night. The fear of missing out (FOMO) plays a major role in this addiction, as mentioned earlier.

Alcohol

Alcohol is insidious, as it denotes a coming of age, the pride of being served in the pub or at the shop, to be able to buy drink for the party or for a friend. From a teen's perspective, it is the ultimate maturity test – to be accepted in a club, pub or off licence! Clearly, it takes a while to become a little resilient to alcohol, and when introduced at a time when we are feeling particularly shy or insecure, we find it gives us our 'Dutch courage', helping us in awkward situations, to overcome our social awkwardness and smooth the way during dinners or parties. This then becomes a lifetime crutch for many who have never learnt to negotiate social situations without alcohol present.

Drugs

Although cannabis is not necessarily chemically addictive, it is habit forming and common among young people, many of whom use it on a weekly if not daily basis. According to research,[2] ketamine, MDMA (3,4-methylenedioxymethamphetamine) and amphetamines are more associated with parties and festive occasions and not necessarily addictive. The area of most concern today is in fact prescribed drugs and how young people sell, give or misuse these drugs on the black market. According to a 2013 paper,[3] in the US (UK trends tend to simulate the US), 'use of prescription opioids and stimulants is a prominent part of the drug abuse problem in the adolescent population'. And according to the Substance Abuse and Mental Health Services Administration (SAMHSA), 'The fastest-growing drug problem in the United States isn't cocaine, heroin, or methamphetamines. It is prescription drugs, and it is profoundly affecting the lives of teenagers.'[4]

Young people seem to have an increasing familiarity with prescription drugs and their use and tend to borrow or buy from each other, in an attempt to either alleviate a condition or to enjoy the tranquillising effects or highs that the drug may give. In a sense, this is more pernicious than illegal drug use as it is socially acceptable and can be continued at the expense of the NHS for their entire lives.

---

2 https://mentoruk.org.uk/get-the-facts

3 Zosel *et al.* 2013.

4 SAMHSA 2017.

Neuroscience of the adolescent brain and addiction (dopamine and addiction)

The neurotransmitter dopamine is an important player in addiction in adolescents, as it is in charge of risk and reward. It rises in the anticipation of an award and has an associated mood enhancement effect. Dopamine is the reason why we do things we like and why they make us happy. So, if we want to feel happy, we want a dopamine reaction. What happens in adolescence is that we need a bigger hit to get the reward. It is evolution's way of making us go out and take risks and leave the village to find a mate! However, if we introduce psychoactive drugs into the picture, the fragile development of the neurotransmitters becomes changed forever, particularly in relation to reward and satisfaction in general life. In time, our sense of satisfaction for the smallest things is no longer present, and moreover, what may be worse, we don't have a memory of being an adult who is satisfied without a drug. This makes it particularly difficult to change the habit later on as we don't have an idea of what things were like before the use of the drug, whether prescription or illegal.

Yoga and addiction

So maybe by now you have some idea how yoga might help with addiction, if we are happy to accept the premise that addiction comes from one or several of the following reasons:

- changes in dopamine in the brain
- need to dull pain
- need to dull anxiety
- need to dull sense of loneliness and separation
- need to cope with chaos.

We know from several studies, over the years, that serotonin levels and GABA levels rise in meditation practices.[5] (Serotonin is a neurotransmitter in the brain associated with joy and pleasure – its absence is an indicator of depression – and GABA is an

5 Krushnakumar, Hamblin and Lakshmanan 2015.

anti-anxiety neurotransmitter.) The most exciting outcome of many research trials and anecdotal evidence is that the neural pathways in the brain are always changing, and in yoga they change in optimal ways, allowing for more connectivity and optimal neurotransmitter levels.

The long-term goal of yoga is of connection, to feel oneness with others in the room, others on the planet and the universe itself, through meditation, movement and breath. This is not simply a desired visualisation but many people's lived experience. There are several yoga therapists working exclusively with yoga for addiction, whose expertise has gone into this chapter and who feel strongly that the many facets of yoga support young people out of addiction and into a healthier relationship with life and those around them.

Why do we suffer?

During this chapter I have often mentioned addiction as a way out of suffering, 'to fill the hole inside', so it might be useful here to mention the *kleshas* – the reasons for suffering according to yoga.

The *kleshas* (afflictions) are simply wrong perceptions. They cause suffering during our lifetime and turn everything around. There are five of them:

1. *Avidya* – ignorance is the misconception that what we think is true; this *klesha* is at the root of all the others. *Example*: We believe that we are good at a particular subject, so our whole world crumbles when we get a bad grade in it, as part of our identity has been brought into question. Any statement about who we are is usually wrong. The solution to this is to accept that we might be wrong.

2. *Asmita* – is the misconception that I am the ego. This self-image is not us. *Example*: 'I am poor', 'I am right', 'I am a bad person', and then we trap ourselves in this projection. It becomes a wonderful liberation when we can say 'maybe I'm not right', 'maybe I don't have to be poor', 'maybe this is not me'.

3. *Raga* – is the attraction to things that bring satisfaction; the sweet taste on the end of the tongue soon becomes a bitter taste, the falling in love soon becomes a daily struggle.

Example: We are attracted to sweets; we think the more we get the more satisfied we will become, but soon we realise we just feel sicker and sicker until we get cavities in our teeth and get fat!

4. *Dvesha* – is the aversion towards unpleasant experiences. We don't want to suffer, yet sometimes in life it is the unpleasant experiences that teach us the most. *Example*: I don't like working hard, it is boring, and I'd rather be out with my friends.

5. *Abinivesha* – is the most universal *klesha* and is the will to live. *Example*: We suffer because we are afraid of death. However, it is precisely when a dear friend or family member dies that we recognise the value of life itself. Death can be a wonderful reminder to live life fully.

'Addicted people often feel incomplete, inadequate and worthless. They want to alleviate these feelings, but addictive behaviour is counterproductive. It brings only more dissatisfaction and emptiness in the long term.' Swami Sivananda shows insight into this perennial problem.[6]

What does this mean to us today? How can we describe this in a meaningful way to young people?

An important part of these lessons or sessions will be the sharing, so developing a sense of connection, caring and support.

When we have found something that works to dull the pain or repress a memory, it means it is working – why would we want to change? But when we see the destructive aspect of the addiction, we need to replace the addiction with something that will work just the same – it is essential that this takes the time it takes and there is no rushing.

Exercises to counter addiction

1. Check in – question how's things, how was the week (don't expect any massive revelations, this is just an opportunity to open up and relax and feel a connection).

6 Sivananda 2004, p.23.

2. *Vinyasa* flows are good as they take the mind off rumination and require concentration, so you could start with the sun salutation, really accentuating the strong holds.

3. Deep relaxation between postures is important; be patient and know that this will take time for them to deeply relax and trust.

4. Try some simple balancing postures – also good for concentration and focus – maybe flows with balancing (example – warrior two, warrior three, tree, dancer and then on the other side).

5. Forward bends for comfort – so coming into child posture with soothing music – invite them to take some deep breaths and maybe move intuitively to release shoulders, back and sides. Maybe come into cat cow if that feels appropriate. Emphasise soothing oneself.

6. If the scenario allows, practise a visualisation of the five bodies:

   - Bringing awareness to the physical body – tensing and releasing throughout (about five minutes).

   - Bringing awareness to the breath, in and out (about three minutes).

   - Bringing awareness to mind, watching the thoughts flow in and out, becoming the witness to the thoughts, noticing them like a dream or a movie, not getting involved (three minutes).

   - Bringing awareness to intellect (notice the critical mind, the judgements and values that you have – this one is tricky and might take some time).

   - Bringing awareness to a light beneath all these layers that shines through, like a light inside a lampshade. Notice it permeates all the other layers like sunshine through the leaves.

7. Bringing awareness back to breath and breath in unison – extending the outbreath and also *ujjayi* to soothe.

8. Finish with a short, light sharing.

— Chapter 13 —

SOCIAL ISOLATION

For your journal

How do we become socially isolated?

How does that make us feel – have you ever felt socially isolated and alone?

What is connection?

What is belonging?

How do we create a sense of belonging in a yoga class?

I changed school at sixth form because I felt I had outgrown my secondary school, I was fed up with the strict Catholic values and the old friends and all the drama. I was ready for something new. But I didn't realise how hard it was going to be. Everyone was already in their friendship groups. I joined the football team and that was good, but they were all about going out and getting drunk after the match. I went along, because I wasn't really having much of a social life, so I thought I might as well. But after a pizza and a few beers, they would go to a club and there would be all these people there, taking drugs and getting drunk and then taking photos. I tried it for a while, but then I thought, no, this isn't for me. I went home and started playing my guitar more and getting on with my homework. Can't lie, it was a pretty lonely time. But, thankfully, I started to meditate at home and did some exercises and online I found others who were into that kind of thing and we started to hang out. The meditation kind of calmed me down and made me realise it wasn't such a big deal and the yoga we did together made me

> realise that I wasn't such a freak or a geek, it's just I didn't want to self-destruct! (Josh, 17)

What is social isolation?

Social isolation is defined by feeling left out and alone. I have had many students in transition, usually Year 7 (11–12-year-olds) or 12 (16–17-year-olds) or first year at university, who struggle with adapting to the new circumstances. First, there is the new ethos of the school, college or university. Each institution has its own set of rules and ways of thinking and being that differ wildly, and it takes time to adapt. Second, leaving dramas behind, we sometimes also leave good friendships and well-known infrastructure behind; we miss the human architecture of a familiar territory which is soothing and supportive to growth and stability. Third, adapting to the new level of education and all its demands, moving from primary school to secondary is a shock for most pupils, as is from secondary to sixth form, where tutors and teachers expect a far greater level of autonomy and engagement from the student than before. Similarly, for university students, the transition to university often entails living by themselves for the first time, which brings its own issues.

Being socially isolated can be depressing and anxiety-inducing for most people. We are social animals, especially during the time of adolescence, as we have stated, when we are actively looking to participate in the world around us.

Isolated in connection

We are born literally connected to our mother through the umbilical cord; we spent the first nine months of life inside another human being. Until we are 13 months, we cannot truly understand separation, it is anathema to our experience thus far in life. In yoga we learn that we are all one; separation is an illusion. Some of the research in addiction shows that the main driver for many addicts is the desire to belong and to connect. The drug gives them a sense of belonging to a blissed state, to connection and love. How do drugs do this? By slowing down the mind. Most drugs flood the brain with endorphins, thus slowing down the critical intellect and favouring the feeling of connection. In *tantra*, this is sometimes referred to as the practice of (metaphorically) cutting off the head to honour the heart. When we move away from our chattering, wandering mind, we come into a state of no-mind, the Buddhist's ideal state. The ego separates, the heart heals and brings together.

Subtle aspects of connection

Social media encourages the photo, the material aspect of our 'selves' portrayed, projected out to the world, to get as many likes as possible. What is this doing to our sense of belonging? On the face of it we are connecting with people worldwide; we find friends who share our point of view, our passion and our hate. We feel empowered, connected. But our physical experience is of being alone. There is more than meets the eye in connection. There are hormones that are constantly speaking to each other, person to person, there are subtle eye and hand movements that all have meaning and are instrumental in how connected or close we feel to certain people. On social media we are reduced to opinion and looks, disembodied, as it were, from our full expression. We have recently noticed a correlation between poor mental health and the sense of isolation and also with increased time on social media. It seems clear to me that if a yoga teacher is able to create a safe, comfortable space where we are encouraged to accept ourselves and each other with compassion and honesty, it would be a positive counterbalance to the disjointing world of social media. Social media is here to stay – it is as much part of young people's lives as TV was for the generation of the 1970s; it forms an inherent part of communication, friendship, courtship and information research. The question is how we deal with it, counterbalance it and use it in a constructive and helpful way.

> I used to get sad when people were mean but now, after doing the yoga, I don't care what other people think of me, I know I'm a good person. (Felipe, 13)

Belonging to oneself, belonging to community

As previously stated, the aim of yoga is to become aware of our oneness with all around us. The word yoga means exactly that – union – union with others, with our world, with our environment and with ourselves. What does it mean to be internally unified?

In the ancient yoga texts it is explained that the *ahamkara* (ego) has as one of its main functions the task of separating us; it means, literally, the I-maker. This is the part of the brain (together with three others) that separates us from the outside world. The more active this part of us is, the more separate we feel. However, the three other parts of the mind, the *buddhi*, the *chitta* and the *manas*, all have different roles to help us to come to a state of transcendence, reached by the activity of the *buddhi* (hence the name Buddha), which is a discriminatory function of the mind and leads us to deep wisdom.

To feel unity within oneself entails sublimating the ego, and realising its proper place in the mind, as a ladder towards greater discrimination and eventually towards a visceral experience of oneness.

Unfortunately, such deep insight and curiosity of the workings of the mind is not common today. Instead we remain in the ego, spending inordinate amount of time creating the I – even to the point of creating an online brand, an online identity, which shows the attractive aspects but deletes anything undesirable.

These activities do not bring us closer to ourselves but rather take us into the realm of creating a false identity. Belonging to ourselves, we travel in the opposite direction; we go inwards, towards the heart of the matter, towards a wilderness that is unchartered and pure.

When we belong to our self, we allow ourselves to be, compassionately and kindly; we turn inwards and sit with our pain, our suffering and our joy, tending to the garden of our heart. When we are able to truly sit with ourselves in harmony and kindness, then this can be taken outwards when others come into view. We are on the path towards showing up 100 per cent for whoever we meet.

When we are seen in this authentic light, letting the mask fall and accepting the human being in front of us as much as we accept the human inside, then we can feel a true belonging. For many the yoga community is the place that this can happen for the first time.

Exercises to increase the sense of belonging, through introspection

These exercises can be done in groups or individually.

1. Focus on the unified movement and breath in the room.
2. Go through the sun salutation in harmony, making sure everyone is moving in sync, like a dance, led by the breath.
3. Partner yoga: around 5–6 postures that you demonstrate, and then get them to make one up.
4. Mandalas (group postures).

   (Please be aware if anyone feels left out, and make sure you are supersensitive to any drama or conflict between partners and change them quickly if so. You might even like to change after each posture to avoid any potential old conflict arising.)
5. End with a relaxation in the round, heads in the middle, maybe hands touching, if it feels right, breathing in unison, visualising light shining on everyone and connecting everyone, everyone's breath entering the trees, the trees breathing them...
6. Group river of oms – everyone is hugging, with an inner and an outer circle, if there are lots of you and everyone just does their sound of om; if someone doesn't want to om or if someone is feeling particularly vulnerable, let them stand in the middle, it can be an amazing experience.
7. Singing together.

— Chapter 14 —

BULLYING

For your journal

Have you ever been bullied?

Have you ever bullied someone?

Why do people bully?

Do you think there has been a shift in perspective around bullying?

How do we respond to a bully in a compassionate and effective way?

Three male students came into my yoga class – they came before the others and there was clearly history between two of them versus the third, who was being very defensive. The aggressors were very subtle in their aggression to start with; not much was needed to intimidate Angus, the third person. It was chilling to watch how a look or a movement brought terror to Angus's face as he physically looked for a safe space in the room. He walked towards me and engaged me so as to be able to ignore the other two. I could tell this ugly dance had been going on for years. They were 14 at this stage. After years of teaching in schools, what I saw unfold with the help of the yoga practice over the next few weeks was quite beautiful and memorable. Initially I just observed the dynamic, carefully placing Angus in the room in such a way that he was separated from the other two and also separating the two from each other, thereby dissipating their power. What we did worked like a dream and has been successful in several different situations since, and I have shared it with you below in the practical section.

What is bullying?

Bullying is when someone harangues and hassles another to the point of despair. Bullying has been an intrinsic part of society for centuries. The public school system has long accepted the method of 'ragging', taunting, ridiculing and teasing. The famous depiction of this is in William Golding's *Lord of the Flies*,[1] where a group of young boys are brought together, and the common denominator is the fight for power through ragging until the boys are distraught and destroyed by each other's cruelty. The victim is often one who is open, vulnerable and maybe smaller in stature than the others.

Why do bullies feel the need to bully? What need does it fulfil in them?

Could it be the need for respect and recognition? Could it be the need to feel important and powerful? Could it be the need for connection through any means possible? I spoke to a group of young men who suggested that sometimes the reason for bullying behaviour is that secretly the bully is jealous of the person who is seen to be a nerd or a geek, as they are so completely themselves. The person who is at the receiving end of the bullying can sometimes be someone who is unapologetically themselves. This is perceived as threatening as it is an empowering and impressive state to those who are desperate to fit in. Often the bully themselves has low self-esteem or low confidence or feels unloved or vulnerable and is keen to make sure no one sees or notices their vulnerability. They need to feel the group behind them – they need to feel belonging to continue being the perpetrator. However, the cost they pay is to hide their own true nature behind the mask of tyranny.

How do we help the bully to stop?

Traditionally, schools try to nip any bullying in the bud, with various punishments. However, these are often counter-productive, as the victim becomes even more victimised for grassing on them, so fuelling the vicious circle to keep on turning. If the bully is acting in a specific way because of their own vulnerability, then making them feel accepted and safe may well be a helpful way to support them in coming away from destructive behaviour for themselves, their peers and society in the long run. If we can encourage them to

1 Golding 1954.

drop the mask, even for a minute or so in relaxation, we have invited them to be more present with their own authentic self, opening the door to a more satisfying experience of relationship and belonging. Bullying behaviour can go on through into adulthood.

How do we support the young person who is being bullied?

Working in a school, it can be easy to point out the ones who will be targeted by the bullies, as they have a vulnerable air about them. Maybe they like being by themselves, or they have some kind of disability. Recently, I have noticed a general trajectory towards a greater level of acceptance of sexual orientation, racial difference and disabilities, often due to tolerance taught at primary school.

Bullying has also taken on a very different profile and dimension through social media. Outside of the teachers and parents' horizon lies an entire world of communication, open to second-by-second cyberbullying. We have all heard of incidents where boys and girls are driven to self-harm or even suicide because of the experience of social isolation, driven by a group of bullies. The recent advent of anonymous social media can make bullying even more pernicious as we are able to divorce ourselves completely from our actions and words. These apps work in such a way that we can post an anonymous, untraceable comment on a timeline – these can be either flattering or bullying.

How do we understand bullying in the context of yoga?

Referring back to the main tasks of adolescence, we remember that belonging to a group is one of the main desires and necessities, in order to move from the family and come into a healthy transitional phase of separation and distance. However, sometimes the cost is great. Maybe we 'get into the wrong crowd', where the modus operandi is to alienate others in order to raise ourselves up, or to define ourselves by who is in and who is out of the group, or to define power by diminishing others.

As we have mentioned previously, the ultimate goal of yoga is the lived experience of union, oneness with ourselves and with our community and world. If, with the practice of yoga, we can offer this lived experience, then the need to isolate, reject and control others becomes less intrinsic. In fact, once this is experienced, then we only want to find ways of experiencing that again and again, as, conversely, this is exactly what we wanted in the first place by creating a defined group of people.

On a more concrete note, the actual yoga class becomes its own context (*sangha*) family, social group, striving towards equanimity, *sattwa* and inclusion, which in itself would counter bullying. Increased compassion for oneself and therefore others would also necessarily lead to the inability to harm or want to harm another.

I remember speaking to an Ofsted officer once who had been sent to inspect two schools in Lancashire. He said, with wonder, that they had exactly the same catchment area, same number of students and same timetable but for one difference, that one of them started the day with meditation. This school showed better overall results, reported little or no antisocial behaviour and in fact was happy to receive 'tricky' students into the fold. This got me thinking and I did some research to find details about the Maharishi Free School in Lancashire, founded in 1986, which is a non-academically selective school. It had overall a good rating by Ofsted on its last inspection in 2013, offers education to 4–15-year-olds and has recently refused to offer SATs (statutory assessments) to students in defence of their mental health. In 2002 the *Liverpool Daily Post* reported that the school had a 100 per cent pass rate on GCSE tests in seven out of the prior eight years. It appears that the Maharishi School was in fact outstanding in many categories and had excelled both academically and in terms of mental health and prosocial behaviour among its pupils.

We can only assume that if a school is willing to offer yoga on a weekly basis to its students and staff (as a whole school approach) then we would probably see similar benefits as those derived from the daily meditation practice at the Maharishi School.

How could yoga and mindfulness help stop bullying?

When we invite our young people to be with themselves in silence with kind and loving guidance, we invite introspection and kindness. We invite compassion to whatever is in this moment, whether there is annoyance, jealousy, hatred or anger. In our increasing compassion to the body we learn to overcome aggression towards ourselves and finally for others.

We learn a dual focus of awareness, we are able to see ourselves or another in the centre of whatever drama is unfolding. This leads to compassion and empathy. Also, as we down-regulate our stress mechanism, and come into the parasympathetic nervous system, we are no longer vigilant and defensive, but rather accepting and prosocial.

Exercise to combat bullying

To combat bullying we need to accentuate connection, community, compassion and empathy.

This starts with our own body.

1. As they are lying on the floor, get them to scan any areas of tension or pain in the body, whether internal or external. Maybe even invite them to scan their minds – memories, reflections or projections – and see if there is any tension there. If there is, invite them to breathe into that space and release the tension, visualising it melting into the floor.

2. As you do your warm up, do the same, accentuating that they take their time with each posture and feeling into it, so if there is a posture or a particular part of the warm up that feels particularly good to them, they can linger there a while.

3. Encourage deep introspection throughout the practice, to allow them to feel into themselves.

4. Come into power postures, such as crow, warrior, really deeply engaging the major muscle groups and accentuating their feeling of power. Be very aware about not going too far, as this might have the opposite effect of disheartening those who are not very accomplished yet – I find the combination warrior three, warrior one and heron in the nest to be perfect for the first time. You can progress to hand stands, crow and bird of paradise as they get more proficient. Encourage

compassion and support for each other; praise should be quiet and individual and targeting those who have a good attitude.

5. Then bring them into partner postures again, changing partner often if there is any kind of tension between partners. Focus on them feeling into their own tension and then checking in with their partner.

6. The more trust is developing, the trickier partner postures you can do, eventually coming into acroyoga.

7. As you progress, invite them to really feel into the other's experience, what hurts for them, how you can make it better for them...

8. *Metta* meditation goes well here:

   May I be well and joyful.
   May I be healthy and at ease.
   May I meet challenges with determination and courage.

   Start by directing this mantra outwards towards your friends and family, then those you don't know very well, then finally to yourself.

9. End with a relaxation which accentuates dropping the mask, feeling into one's own power and being a force for good.

Suggested script: Letting go of the body into the mat, become aware of your breath, that you share with every living creature. Allow your awareness to rest at the centre of your body, in the heart. Follow the beat of your heart as it slows down during this relaxation and as the breath deepens. Feeling the body relax and let go, as the power of your heart connects you with your own courage and life force. Know the power you have within yourself to forge ahead in all circumstances. Know that you have wisdom deep inside your heart which guides you to your best possible destiny, choosing love over hate and choosing expansion over contraction. Let go of any expectations you might have of yourself in this moment, just for a minute, let go of any judgement or preconception, allowing the present moment to be just as it is. Knowing that your breath is the connection between this body and your life, the rock which you can always connect with, allowing the mind to settle into the heart. The breath deepens and takes you on an inward journey into the heart, the centre of wisdom, light and power. Rest here for a few moments. Know you are enough. Drop the mask of who you think you ought to be and rest in the knowledge that you are enough. Imagine what it might feel like to be enough, to drop expectations of yourself and others, just being in your own heart right now. (After a few minutes, judge for yourself.) Now take a deep breath, raising the chest, and as you exhale start to move the fingers and toes, remaining still inside. Thank yourself for deeply resting and know that this is always available to you. Wiggle your toes and fingers and roll over onto your right side before you get up.

— Chapter 15 —

RELATIONSHIPS

For your journal

Did you have a best friend?

Did you find friendships easy?

Did you feel you belonged to a group?

How did you get together with your first partner?

He was my only friend, so when he asked me to come and witness for him in court, I didn't want to let him down, I wanted to do the right thing. I was there on the night she said she'd been raped. I knew it was a lie. I couldn't tell my folks, 'cos they'd kill me, going to court and that. I mean, do I get a criminal record? I dunno. So I went and, man, they treated me like I was a rapist, I mean I only went to help my mate out! It was not nice. But he got off the hook and that's the main thing; she told me after that she'd just said that 'cos she didn't want her folks to know she was seeing this other bloke and that's why she was pregnant. (Caz, 16)

Patanjali wrote:

Maitrikaruna muditopekshanam
sukhadukhapunyapunyavishayanam bhavanataschitta
prasadanam

By practising the habits of friendliness, compassion, happiness and virtues and by being indifferent to misery and sinful vices, your mind is pleasant. (Patanjali Yoga Sutra #33)

Explanation:

> When we are friendly towards happy people and have a feeling of inclusion, we will not be jealous. With unhappy people, have compassion, but do not be friendly as it drags you down. With people who seem lucky, who have good grades, good jobs, be happy for them (help them and learn from them). With people who are doing wrong acts, ignore them, do not judge, do not linger.

Getting on with people

Future success in life is often dependent on getting on well with people. How we relate to the world around us is shaped by a variety of factors. At the very base of it is our world view – do we live in a predominantly optimistic inner world or is it negative? Do we trust or do we not? What formed our world view and how can it change to support a peaceful existence? If we do, in fact, completely adhere to the basic meaning and therefore philosophy of yoga, which is that all is one and we are all one, then a relationship is simply one part of us relating to another part of us, like a hand relates to the other hand or an arm to the shoulder – we are all in it together and nothing can tear us apart; all division and separation is completely illusory.

If we can find our way to a healthy attachment, in a trusting mindset, where our fellow human beings are our supporters and collaborators rather than our competitors, it stands to reason that we will live in a more harmonious world.

Given that we treat others the way we inwardly treat ourselves, it is our first duty to take care of our inner life through such practices as yoga and meditation.

> *Before, I was a nervous kid, I used to insult my friends and defy them, but since I started meditation, it seems I started calming down. I am like another person. I feel more relaxed, freer.* (Carlos, 14)

Friendship

Given that one of the main tasks of adolescence is to move away from parents and family, friendship becomes so much more important than ever before. For some, friendship and making friends is an entirely intuitive and natural process, developing from primary school playdates, sports teams and neighbourhood connections. For others, especially those on the autistic spectrum, friendship is tricky, complicated and unfathomable. It is a question of understanding relatively subtle signals, usually imperceptible to the eye, which indicate whether to come closer or to back off, whether to include or exclude. For many there is a natural anthropologically fixed progression from hanging out in large (sometimes single gender) groups, to moving into smaller interest groups (music, sports, yoga), to pairing off into friendships.

Belonging to a social circle is important for our self-esteem and our identification process that is underway at this time. (Identification: belonging to a group, knowing 'who I am' in relation to society – finding an identity that is optimal to the place where I live.) Sometimes the price is very high. When the norm is to party, have sex, drink or take drugs and you are not comfortable in this scene, it can feel alienating and lonely to pull away from the people that give you a context in which to belong. The teenage years put a lot of pressure on us to conform in order to belong; it takes a secure and strong individual to pull away and enjoy their solitude.

Friendship and yoga

My experience of yoga circles has always been very positive – a group of supportive friendships who are concerned for my wellbeing and my success as much as I am for theirs. We support each other's courses and support each other emotionally through tricky times, we offer free respites to each other and send students to each other, so that they get the best therapist for them. It is a selfless and nurturing group of (mostly) women. I have also noticed that in some contexts, where I have worked, we have managed to create a small, friendly and supportive group of yogis, who have a good influence on each other. They help each other navigate the trickier aspects of teenage life, offering a respite from drugs, sex and relationship confusion.

Intimate relationships and sex

When young people access porn as a precursor to sex, it might well be robbing them of childhood and equally of a mutually satisfying sex life further down the line, believing that they have to live up to the images they have seen. It is only when young people are encouraged to develop an inner life full of reflection and intuition that we have a chance of developing an immunity to this kind of impact. Ideally, we would guide young people away from the desire to look at porn simply through compassion both for themselves and for the people on the screen.

When self-respect and self-esteem are present, porn cannot live side by side with it. Porn is by its very nature violent and misleading, diminishing loving relationships to nothing more than a physical act, which divorces itself from what young people are in fact looking for, which is intimacy, tenderness and belonging.

So how can yoga support healthy intimacy and eventually a healthy sex life?

A healthy sex life is connected to creativity, self-expression, caring and connection. For many women, sex is something that works best when we are relaxed and feel good about our bodies. When we are tense or too preoccupied with what others think of us, we cannot feel true pleasure or ask for what we want in order to feel good.

But in asana we learn where our boundaries are, what feels good and what is too much or too little, we learn to have that inner dialogue with ourselves that we can take into the sex act. We are also learning how to connect the various emotions and feelings in different parts of the body. Similarly, with breathing techniques and relaxation exercises, we become more available to letting go and being spontaneous with our partner.

As a healthy friendship is built on respect, consideration, care and compassion, we can focus on these core principles in our class. We start with building these in our own selves and then go on to build them in relation to others.

Asana exercises

Start off with some classic partner postures for about 20 minutes, exploring with different members of the group. Finally, see if they can create a new partner posture themselves or even a series of postures that flow together.

Self-massage and massage of each other in a circle

Mandala exercises

Everyone stands in a circle in tree posture and you raise your hands up to support and try to push each other over, then come down in forward bend; with hands still touching, come back up. Back right up so that everyone is standing close together in a circle, all facing the same direction, then attempt to sit back on each other, everyone holding each other up. Lie down and have the next person lie down on your stomach, and create a zigzag ladder of people, each laying on the other's stomach – a lovely way to connect; if they giggle, all the better!

Meditation exercise

Finish off with a heart meditation. Get each pair to sit together, one cross-legged and the other facing on knees; both close their eyes. Both have hands on their knees. Take a few breaths here. The kneeling person feels into their own heart and empties themselves in order to become a conduit of light and love. The other prepares to receive. Thinking only positive thoughts or just light, each sits quietly, while the kneeler places both hands either side of the chest of their partner and the other keeps still. It is important that the kneeling one feels themselves a conduit of light, through the head and into the hands, and the other one receives the energy. Keep repeating these instructions; the hands should be in front of and behind the heart, probably in the air. Stay like this for around five minutes and then swap – no chatting and minimal movement. End with a hug.

Group exercises

Coming into the centre, we can do the om circle, where you have an inner circle for those who are feeling tired, vulnerable or otherwise and then an outer circle for those who are feeling stronger. Huddle in really tight and start omming, not necessarily together and not necessarily on the same note (if you can't om for any reason, you can just hum). Carry on doing this for a few minutes.

Now turning the other way, still one inner circle and one outer circle, do eye gazing.

Have a singing bowl or cymbals, and everyone is standing facing someone – when the cymbals go they move to their left; the circle in the middle stays where it is. This needs to move quite fast, as it is very difficult for some people. You can go round twice, if it feels appropriate.

— Chapter 16 —

SLEEP

For your journal

How did your sleep patterns change when you started doing yoga?

How did you sleep as a teen?

How do the teens in your life sleep?

What hampers your sleep?

How does sleep affect your day/mood/character?

When I was younger I walked in my sleep, often finding myself on the landing. I used to have terrible nightmares, I would wake up screaming, such a vivid imagination. I hated going to sleep and would put it off in case I had nightmares. My parents tried to help, but nothing worked. The weed, it helped me get to sleep, I felt my body relax and my mind would slow down, stop the worrying, until I just drifted off, often without dreams. Problem was I would sleep for so long, sometimes missing school, then I noticed my sleep became really erratic, I don't know why, but I do know that I couldn't go to sleep sometimes until 4 in the morning, then of course it was punishing to get up at 7, so I just missed the first periods and came in at lunch or later. So sometimes I tried to just stay up, but then I'd fall asleep as soon as I got home from school and sleep through till the next morning, missing dinner and homework. When I started with the yoga, it was good, I was never the sporty type, so the postures weren't really my thing, but the relaxation bit at the end and some of the breathing really helped me. Now

> I use that at home and I've stopped with the weed. It's getting better, and my rhythms seem to be more regular now. (AS, 20)

Why sleep is so important

In 2017 the NHS reported a dramatic increase in under-14s admitted to hospital for sleep disorders, from 3000 in 2004–2005 to 8000 in 2015–2016.[1] Kathryn Orzech and colleagues say that teens need 9.5 hours' sleep per night and on average only get 7.5.[2] It is believed that screens are the culprit. The blue light that is emitted from screens emulates daylight and therefore play havoc with our melatonin levels. Some say that three-quarters are affected by bad sleep, which, the report shows, contributes to illnesses such as sore throats, obesity, colds, flu and gastroenteritis. I have also noticed that mental health issues are exacerbated by lack of sleep. Moreover, parties and screen time shift sleep patterns away from the natural circadian rhythm, causing a kind of jetlag. A regular rhythm is important for wellbeing in general but it all starts with the sleep pattern. When we allow our bodies to fall into step with nature's own cycles, it works in our favour, getting the most of sunlight's vitamin D during the day and benefiting from the secretion of certain hormones (melatonin versus cortisol) to support healthy and deep sleep. One of the world's foremost yoga researchers also happens to be a professor of sleep medicine at Harvard University. Sat Bir Khalsa states clearly that sleep is a biological need and that sleep disorders come in three main categories: parasomnias (general sleep disruptions), disorder of excessive daytime sleep and insomnia.[3] What we are coming across among teenagers is a case of self-restricted sleep, either because of studying, partying or tech use. A 2015 review paper in the *Journal of Sleep Medicine* by Hale and Guan suggests screen time is adversely associated with sleep outcomes in 90 per cent of studies.[4] According to Dr Khalsa, there are many consequences of self-restricted sleep on an ongoing basis, and these may include:

- cognitive/academic performance impairment

---

1 Kleeman and Drury 2017.
2 Orzech, Salafsky and Hamilton 2011.
3 Khalsa and Butzer 2016.
4 Hale and Guan 2015.

- emotional function and social functioning (being present)
- glucose regulation impairment
- increased appetite and risk for obesity
- increased risk of hypertension
- immune function impairment
- elevated psychophysiological arousal.

Below is a graph on the prevalence of insomnia among young people in Norway.

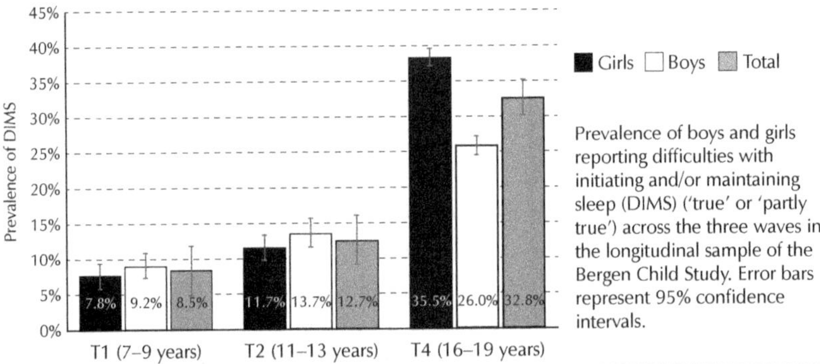

Prevalence of boys and girls reporting difficulties with initiating and/or maintaining sleep (DIMS) ('true' or 'partly true') across the three waves in the longitudinal sample of the Bergen Child Study. Error bars represent 95% confidence intervals.

From Sivertsen, B., Harvey, A.G., Pallesen, S., Hysing, M., Trajectories of sleep problems from childhood to adolescence: A population-based longitudinal study from Norway. *Journal of Sleep Research* (in press).

A major contributing factor to the occurrence and maintenance of insomnia, according to Dr Khalsa, is hyperarousal. The stress response systems, including the sympathetic nervous system, and stress hormones, including adrenaline and cortisol, tend to be elevated in their activity, thereby keeping psychophysiological arousal higher and inhibiting sleep.

One of the conclusions of a paper in *Psychosomatic Medicine* is that 'treatments for insomnia, such as relaxation, exercise training and some medications...may provide long-term benefits over and above short-term improvement in reported sleep quality'.[5]

The following graphs show the impact of yoga on sleep, on both quality and the ability to fall asleep.

5 Hall *et al.* 1998.

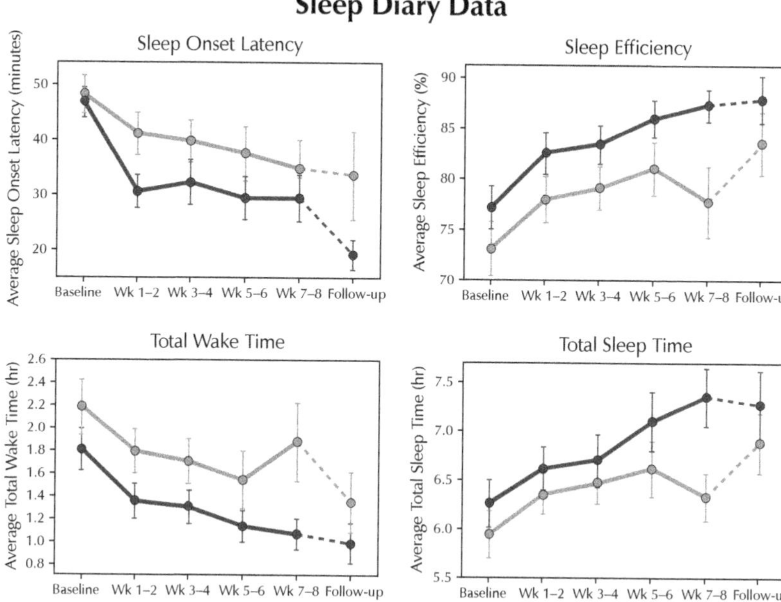

A typical response of a 15-year-old female: 'Yoga definitely helped with sleeping...it would take me a long time to get to sleep. When I was doing yoga it was much easier to fall asleep and stay asleep.'

Sleep and exhaustion

Sometimes we see young people who are truly exhausted but still can't sleep – seems like an oxymoron, but actually it is simply a continuation of the above. The exhaustion is a result of high cortisol levels, never switching off, which do not in fact help sleep. If we continuously fail to honour the correct circadian rhythms we pass the moment of drowsiness and the body will excrete hormones to keep you awake, thereby upsetting the fine-tuned balance of the sleep cycle. We can bring the *gunas*[6] into the equation here and see that, when *rajas* has been too active, we come into *tamas* after a while; this lethargy is not necessarily the *guna* that is the most

6 *Gunas* are the three states of being in nature and in humans, consisting of *tamas*, *rajas* and *sattwa*. All aspects of nature take on one of these qualities at any one time; they can be used to describe people, food, music or situations. *Rajas* denotes a noisy, energetic quality, whereas *tamas* is laziness, lethargy, lack of energy. *Sattwa* is a pure state of harmony and balance.

efficient for you to have a deep and nourishing sleep. The body needs to catch the circadian rhythm just right, hitting it at 10 pm when the body is at its optimal state for sleep, then awake around 6 am when the cortisol helps you to get out of bed; this way you will encourage optimal performance through the day and also stave off both mental and physical illness.

The more we fall into a simple, natural rhythm with nature, in line with *sattwa*, the easier it is to stay well.

The insomnia epidemic

For many young people, FOMO, the fear of missing out, drives them to stay up later than their parents think, to keep online, if they have tablets or phones in their bedrooms. FOMO is particularly strong for the younger teens, from around 13 onwards, who are lulled into the perception that everyone is having amazing lives and they are just boring and excluded from it. To be switched on to people from all over the world in different time zones creates a hunger to know what they are up to or to follow a particular dialogue online, in which, if you left, you might be targeted or mentioned.

I can only imagine how hard it is, when we are at the stage of wanting to fit in and belong, to let go of these moments and to feel OK just being all by oneself. The time when we definitely are left alone is when our parents or carers are asleep, and we then have to get up for school, so naturally our sleep becomes deprived.

Tyranny of time and money

Sometimes it can seem that most of our motivations are based on greed and efficiency, as opposed to acting for the general good and creating quality products, relationships or connections. It is easy to lose ourselves under the tyranny of time and clutched in the iron grasp of greed. Maybe yoga could show us a way out of this, which allows us to connect with something deep inside us – peace, tranquillity, purpose and meaning, which puts the desire for money and the pressure of time in their rightful place.

In terms of finding a way to help students come into sleep we focus on reducing the cortisol, coming into a healthy circadian rhythm and bringing the body out of forced *rajas* or enforced *tamas*, back into *sattwa*. When we are in *sattwa* our intuition will naturally guide us into a place where we know what our body needs.

Yoga knits the ravelled sleeve of care: exercises to help with sleep

Make sure the room is relatively dark – candles really help, as do some kind of incense or smell, such as lavender or chamomile. You can either spray, roll on or burn these smells. The main focus of this class is release and relaxation. Forward bends have a down-regulating effect on the nervous system and may well aid sleep and the feeling of sleepiness. All the way through encourage *ujjayi* breath and elongating the outbreath.

1. Sitting up:

   - Neck rolls: Rather than the old-fashioned way of rolling the entire head one way and then the other, you can simply stretch the head one way and then the other, releasing the side of the neck down to the shoulder. Then move on to the back of the neck. End with dropping the head back into the hands and opening the mouth, so relaxing the jaw completely.

   - Eye rolls: Release the eyes (often tired from too much computer time) by stretching the eyes to the right and then left and then up and down, then eye rolls all around.

   - Shrug the shoulders and roll them around (often also tense from sitting at desks or at computers).

2. Child's pose: Stretch either side of the body by walking the hands over to one side and then the other, bring knees apart and drop body down towards the floor, releasing hips. (This pose is a familiar pose for many teenagers, remembering what it is to feel small.) Try out a few times with the toes flexed under the buttocks, so releasing tension in the toes and back of the feet, which in turn will have an impact on the fascia of the entire body, specifically the lower back. Accentuate the deep breathing in this posture.

3. Downward dog: It is easy to make a sequence of child's pose to downward dog and back again – moving slowly with the breath, taking time over each posture. As they grow, the hamstrings often tighten, and it can be really nice to just stretch them out briefly before coming back to a kneeling posture.

4. Forward bend: Coming into the standing forward bend here is a nice transition, letting the head and shoulders hang loose towards the floor as they shake out the shoulders and loosen the lower back a little. This can be done with bent knees if they are very stiff.

5. Coming into a pigeon posture, with props if needed, allow your students to lie down for several minutes like this, maybe playing some music; this is a perfect hip opener for those who need to relax and may feel vulnerable in other, more common hip openers. It can also be very helpful for lower back pain.

6. At this point please make the room as dark as you can without freaking them out. If you haven't already, you can put some music on too and spray the room or your hands with lavender so that when you come around you can waft the smell close to them. Be careful with touch at this stage as they might be really relaxing and it might jolt them out of the relaxed state.

7. Legs up the wall: We encourage students to come to the wall, bottom right up against the wall and legs up the wall. Initially they can bend their knees and place their feet on the wall; as they push with the feet the bottom comes off the floor and rises up, making a line from knees to hips to shoulders, and then gently, activating the spine, the back comes gently down to the floor again. In this way we are bringing awareness to the thyroid, the vishuddha chakra, the area of balance, of giving and taking. This can be expressed if the group are open to this; either way, get them to focus on the throat when they are up in the position and breathe *ujjayi* at this time. Finally they come down to rest, with legs up the wall and hands on the stomach; you can encourage

hands on the stomach and eye bags for comfort. Ask them to take a few very deep breaths, extending the outbreath. You might also like to introduce the three-part breath here – beginning with the clavicles, then the chest and finally the stomach, and then reverse it. Some find this breathing technique tricky to do, so keep it simple and remember your main aim is for them to slow their breathing right down and slow their mind.

8. If their feet start tingling they can bring them down into a more comfortable position or come down to *savasana* at the end – I recommend that you use music for this bit as many teens find it disconcerting if you are silent. Make the *savasana* as long as you think you can – in the beginning that would be around three minutes, but you can quickly build to 15 minutes or, in some cases, a full yoga *nidra* of 45 minutes after eight or so weeks. The key is to tell them what is about to happen so that they are fully prepared for the relaxation.

I have had quite some success with this routine. Ask them to continue with at least the legs up the wall at home in the evening. They can use the elongation of the outbreath throughout the exercise. They can also drink limeflower, valerian or chamomile tea and have a hot bath and get to bed before 10 pm, having had plenty of exercise and no screens for two hours before bed.

— Chapter 17 —

EXAM SUCCESS

For your journal

Do you remember exams at school – how did they make you feel?

Did your feelings get in the way of succeeding?

How do you think yoga might help?

'Miss, do you remember me?' a ginger-headed young man popped up, next to me at the supermarket. His face was familiar. I smiled. 'You taught me yoga when I did my GCSEs last year' – oh yes, now I remembered. 'Well, you remember that breathing technique you taught us all – I used it in my exams and it worked!' I remember he was ambitious but found certain subjects really tricky and was predicted Bs and Cs. 'Oh yes,' I remembered. 'How did it go?' I asked, curious to hear his news. 'Miss, I got straight As and 3 A*s!' 'Wow, you must have studied really hard, congratulations!' 'Yes, I did, and I used the breathing to keep me focused – so I just wanted to thank you for that.' He bounced off down the aisle with a cheery wave. My heart sang.

Exams at school

Exams are a fundamental part of every British teenager's life. The pressure to do well at an allotted time in a specific way, to jump through hoops that might lead to some kind of success later on, is a complicated set of thought processes at the best of times, let alone at a time when our prefrontal cortex is playing hide and seek! It seems clear to me from experience as a teacher, but also as a parent, that a calm, collected mind, with optimal emotional support, does better, on average, than one without that scaffolding.

So, if we just break down what happens during exams, we can see how exactly we can support the process with yoga. Passing an exam means planning, focusing in class, being able to keep emotions in check and calming the mind to focus it on your task in hand. On the way, many temptations need to be resisted and the prefrontal cortex will need to do a lot of growing. One of the main issues facing many young people who have difficulty studying is the ability to stay on topic and not wander over a period of two years. The other difficulty for many is the rising interest in sex as well as partying and all that that entails. Remaining grounded and on track is essential and easier for those who have a firm and solid attachment at home or with someone significant in their lives, who can hold and care for them through this tumultuous time. For those who do not have this, I firmly believe that yoga could fulfil that function to some degree, by creating a safe and functioning practice that allows the student to connect deeply with their own calm, that gives them an opportunity to learn about disciplining the mind and the body, and which guides and supports them through life with wisdom.

Exam preparation exercises

Things to do before exams

1. Sleep well (follow steps below).
2. Switch off any screens at least an hour before bed.
3. Don't drink coffee or alcohol or eat sugar after supper (even better, avoid them altogether if you can).
4. Have a hot bath with lavender or chamomile essential oils before bed.
5. Massage yourself slowly with warm almond oil (pop it on the radiator) together with lavender drops (failing that, both almond oil and sesame oil that you get from the food shop

are fine; don't go for vegetable, sunflower or olive oil as they smell pretty bad!).

6. Have a chamomile/limegrass/valerian tea one hour before bed.
7. Eat at regular times and sleep at regular times, bed around 9.30–10 pm and up at around 7 am (teens need 8–10 hours' sleep at night).
8. Make sure your room is cool and clean with fresh air and your bed is warm and clean.
9. Read something inspiring before bed for a few minutes.
10. *Ujjayi* breath for ten minutes in the evening.
11. Eat well (lots of veg, lots of water; not too much sugar, as sugar can cause mental confusion).

Outside the exam hall or just before (exercises designed to be done standing)

1. Focusing breath, *analoma viloma*: Breathe in for the count of four through the left nostril, and out for eight or four, through the right nostril, and then in four right, out eight left – carry on for as long as it is comfortable (5–10 minutes).
2. Breathe in three steps; imagine a ladder – breathe up each rung, one at a time, pause in between and then breathe out *ujjayi* breath (Darth Vader sound, like when you close the back of your throat a bit to make a hissing sound) – do this for about five minutes or more if you like. If you feel dizzy or uncomfortable then stop.
3. Lion's breath, to feel courageous: Tense your whole body and face as you inhale and then let out a roar as you stick out your tongue, open your eyes wide and open hands – do this several times.

Stress-relieving exercises

1. Chair posture (affirmation: I am calm).
2. Twist in chair (affirmation: I am rooted).
3. Warrior (make the bend in the knee deep) (affirmation: I am a warrior).
4. A quick sun salutation, if you have time (affirmation: I am ready).

Focusing exercises

1. Balancing postures – dancer (affirmation: I am focused).
2. Tree (affirmation: I am rooted and balanced).

Tension-release exercises

1. Shoulder release – more dancer or clasping hands on lower back and forward bend, *ujjayi* breath and lift arms as high as they can go.
2. Shoulder rolls.
3. Hip rolls.
4. Hands on hip bones, arch back both ways, cat cow – several times.
5. Side bends with hands above the head – stretch arms above the head, lift the right arm and hand and tip over to the left, hold for a count of ten and do the other side. Once each side, slowly.

Visualisation for exams

Imagine yourself sitting at the desk in the examination hall (acquaint yourself with the hall first if you can). You are completely quiet and still; bring your awareness to the feet – feel as if they have roots in the ground, growing roots downwards, drawing inspiration from Mother Earth – inspiration flowing through you (what does it look like?), calm belly, and a golden light infuses you with wisdom while you confidently fully answer each question. Imagine the clothes you will be wearing, the table, where you will be sitting, the pen you will use and how you feel completely confident. It is good to spend some time working out exactly how it feels to be confident and, if you don't feel confident, imagine you do!

Know that your mind can be your ally or your enemy, depending on you. Which thoughts are you entertaining? We all have thoughts like 'I am not good enough, I am an imposter, I am just faking it'. But we also have thoughts like 'I know this stuff, I am intelligent, I can do this, I have studied hard and I can do my best here and now'.

Which thought is best to choose? If you have difficulty with unwanted thoughts, it can sometimes help to have a song or a mantra in your head that brings you back to a positive state of mind – mine used to be *I Will Survive* by Gloria Gaynor! But nowadays I use an even more positive mantra – om; if you just repeat the sound A-O-U-M with each outbreath quietly in your mind, it will empty your mind a little, then you can refocus.

Top tip: You retain information in rapid eye movement (REM) sleep between 1 am and 4 am – if your sleep is disturbed or not of good quality, you will not remember what was learned!

It is also a *tapas*, to spend time doing something you don't want to do, to enhance your self-discipline. When I started playing the piano, I didn't want to practise, but I did, and now I can play a few pieces. There is always something the mind does not want to do but that eventually it benefits from. Stephen Covey says: 'Can you play the piano? I can't. I don't have the freedom to play the piano. I never disciplined myself… What about the freedom to forgive, to ask forgiveness? What about the freedom to love unconditionally, to be a light, not a judge – a model, not a critic? Think of the discipline involved in these. Discipline comes from being "discipled" to a person or a cause.'[1]

So discipline leads to freedom, every time.

1 Covey 2005, p.74.

Exercises for mapping your sleeping habits and what you eat

Map your sleeping habits in your journal; write down (honestly!) how long you spend on screens and how long there is between switching off your screen and bed time. Map what you eat during a week – how many vegetables and fruit versus sweets and biscuits.

PART III

— Chapter 18 —

SUCCESS

For your journal

How do you define success?

What do you think is the most common definition of success?

What do you believe that you need to sacrifice in order to be successful?

She'd reached the goal, she was sitting in the halls of residence, at the top university of her choice, having aced her A-levels. Her dad had got her an old banger, she was studying her favourite subject. Her boyfriend had got into the same uni. They could go home every weekend if they wanted to. But something was missing, she felt sad inside, disconnected. Her health had deteriorated with all the pressure to get here. Noticing the yoga class, she started taking a class every week to get fit again after the studying and soon noticed her body felt freer, her mind felt calmer and her joy started to return. Her body and mind had paid a price for her success and she wanted to reclaim her health. Within three months she was studying with more focus, allowing for more time for friends and family and her health had improved. She would no longer make choices that impacted on her health.

Common definitions of success

We live in a society that espouses values far from yogic values. Success for some young people today is having money, looks, an attractive partner and an interesting job. We take it for granted that these signify success and therefore joy. Many are surprised and depressed when (if) they attain these goals and still find something is missing for them.

Our entire society is geared towards succeeding in exams, succeeding in getting a job or creating income for oneself, however that is done. I am always struck by the difference, when I teach in Muslim countries, where there is a conscious pull among devout Muslims (of which there are many, maybe the majority), towards spiritual and soul and away from the material world.

So, what do we want to succeed at? I presume that most people want health and happiness. Without these you don't have a meaningful life. So, if success is health and happiness, we need to master these two states. In order to succeed at anything, we need to master it. But how can you master anything, how can you succeed in anything, without understanding it completely?

For your students we can hope that, through these practices, they learn to succeed in life, by mastering themselves, understanding the way their bodies, minds and spirit work. Yoga is skilful action, making enlightened choices, that render your life full, joyful and of service to others, saying yes to life. Mastering yoga is mastering life itself, finding meaning, joy and flow.

Years of wrong thinking around the meaning of success has wreaked havoc with our ecological system, our natural values of care and compassion and in the development of children into responsible, loving adults.

> *Every school is looking for solutions to some major problems. The solutions need to be easy to implement and truly effective. Since yoga has come to our school the students have changed. They can control themselves better, they look more relaxed, focused. They have become more aware of their feelings and emotions.* (Anna Velazquez, Teacher, Spain)

Success in yoga terms

If instead of appearances we focus on our inner state, instead of financial success we focus on moral and ethical success, with our planet at the centre – we may move into a more mindful and supportive world with a beautiful and flourishing future. Each of us has a role in this, and each is different. In the Bhagavad Gita, Arjuna is called upon to act out his dharma – the path that is calling him in this life. The entire story is about how he comes to terms with his role as a warrior. Many of us have callings in this life and come across many struggles before we surrender to the path that is offered to us.

The four principles of dharma are compassion, truth, discipline and purity. Simon Haas (2015) eloquently writes about them in *The Book of Dharma: Making Enlightened Choices*:

> ...each of these four principles needs to be understood and interpreted in relation to the others. Thus, Discipline here refers to focused effort that is also non-violent and grounded in Truth. Likewise, Truth is not a serene state of mind: it must be lived. This entails great Discipline.
>
> The reason we don't manage to invoke Dharma fully is that we don't usually apply all four Dharma principles together. We usually apply just one of them, or at best two. This is like pushing down on the acceleration pedal of a car while simultaneously leaving three handbrakes partially on.
>
> When we want to achieve something, the Dharma principle we tend to reach for immediately is Discipline. In other words, we want to put in as much effort as possible. But if our effort is in the wrong direction, how can it yield an optimal result? Discipline in the Dharma Code is therefore not effort, but 'right effort'. The secret to invoking Dharma in our life is therefore not to apply one of the Dharma principles, but to apply all of them, simultaneously.

All four principles are looked at below.

1 Compassion (ahimsa)

When we speak of compassion, we mean compassion towards ourselves first. Are the relationships you are having healthy and helpful and supportive to your growth? Are they damaging in any way – can that change? Then compassion for others – is there a way in which I could show deeper understanding towards my friends, my family and my school friends?

Ahimsa was the leading principle of Mahatma Gandhi and he managed to initiate independence for India through his peaceful protest!

Exercise about compassion

1. Think of someone you love (not a boyfriend or girlfriend) and send them kindness; imagine smiling at them in the place you normally see them, maybe even giving them a hug.
2. Now move onto someone you like and do the same thing.
3. Next, someone who you don't feel specially anything for and do the same thing.
4. Then move onto a relative and repeat.
5. Then move onto someone you don't know very well at all and repeat.
6. Then imagine someone you don't like very much and imagine smiling warmly at them, sincerely.
7. Finally, imagine meeting yourself and doing this too.

2 Your truth (satya)

In life there is Truth, and your truth. Truth is that the apple falls to the floor if you drop it. Your truth is that you might really like your science teacher but not your French teacher! It has nothing to do with the outside world, or even if you are right or not, it is just your truth.

There is also the truths of all truths, which in Vedanta yoga is that you are the embodiment of Truth, Bliss and Consciousness (God, Universal Energy).

Come out to yourself! Be truthful in your own mind before all else! It is no good pretending to yourself.

As Polonius said in *Hamlet*, Act 1:3:

This above all: to thine own self be true,
And it must follow, as the night the day,

> Thou canst not then be false to any man.
> Farewell, my blessing season this in thee!

As soon as you start to have compassion for yourself, you can no longer lie to yourself, and you gain self-respect. Sometimes we think one thing, say another and act in a third way. This is exhausting and a little bit scary, as you are always worried you are going to get found out! What if you said one thing to your friends, so they would like you, and then you said something different to another person, and they talked to each other?

Unfortunately, truth always comes out in the end! So, before you say something, check in with yourself. Then your words will have so much more power.

Did you hear the story about the mother who wanted her son to stop eating sweets?

> She went to the monk and begged him to tell her son to stop eating sweets, as he was getting fatter and fatter and had so many holes in his teeth! The monk said, 'Unfortunately I can't help you today, please come back in two weeks.' The mother came back and the monk looked at her son and said, 'Stop eating sweets.' Her little son looked up at the monk and never ate sweets again. The mother came back a few weeks later and asked, 'Why didn't you tell him straight away, why did I have to come all the way back here?' The monk said, 'I was eating sweets myself at that time, my words would have had no impact.'

Exercise about your truth

1. Make a note of things you say that you don't mean or that you don't believe but you say so that you can fit in or belong.
2. Notice if you ever think one thing, say another and act in a third way.
3. Are your thoughts, words and actions in alignment?

Don't worry if this happens a lot, it is sometimes very difficult to think, say and act the same thing. It needs a lot of practice, and you need to remember that compassion always comes first!

3 Discipline (tapas)

At first, discipline is no fun for anyone. To be told to do stuff is not easy. But you know that feeling when you have practised something again and again and you see the result, whether it is piano, football, gaming, dance or singing, you get good at whatever you spend your time doing! That is discipline.

Of course, it is easier if you love it and you are good at it.

The famous author Joseph Campbell said 'follow your bliss'. He meant that, if you carry on doing what you love, discipline comes naturally. But sometimes there are times when we need to practise something we are not good at in order to do something we are good at. A pianist may need to practise scales, a footballer may need to run laps, a dancer may need to watch what they eat, all to achieve their goal, to be free to do what they love to do.

Exercise about discipline

1. Can you think of something you love to do, you are quite good at, but feel you are not as good as you could be?
2. What do you need to do to get better at it, to really enjoy it?
3. What would help you to do that?
4. Do it!

4 Purity/cleanliness (saucha), coherence, congruence, alignment

When you translate words from Sanskrit, they often miss an aspect of the meaning. Purity can mean so many things. But it is so refreshing being around someone who tells the truth with love, who is disciplined and clean living, that is, free from clutter.

Is your room full of clothes and stuff that you don't need any more? Could you have a clear out? Are you eating well, or is your body full of unnecessary foods that you don't need any more? Is your mind full of thoughts and worries you no longer need? How about your emotions, are they clear and simple or complicated?

All these things have to do with the word *saucha*, or purity.

Exercise about purity

1. What in your room could you get rid of, give to a friend or to the charity shop?
2. What foods are you eating that are making you feel bloated or constipated?
3. Which thoughts are you having that are unkind or not helpful to you or others?

You will notice how one of these follows on from the next and how they are all connected. You might also notice that, when you start paying attention to these aspects, you will feel compelled to do something about it.

When you have managed to see to these four pillars, your path may well be clear to you in your life, and if not, then simply do your best and keep moving forward and, soon, everything will be revealed!

— Chapter 19 —

HAPPINESS

For your journal

Write down your happiest memory.

Do you remember the last time you saw a happy baby?

What does it make you feel like when someone you love is happy?

Coming out of the yoga class, colours seemed brighter, time seemed like it had slowed down. All the things that had bugged me before I went in seemed to have dropped back into a less important place in my mind. As I jumped on my bike to go home, I seemed to have unlimited energy and flew home. I was truly happy!

The role of happiness

I remember my first yoga theory class at the Sivananda Centre in Putney in 1998 – the teacher turned to the class and asked: 'What does every human being want?'

The answer was – happiness. Everything we do is to attain happiness: when we eat good food, it is because we hope it will make us happy; when we spend time with our friend, it is to make us happy; when we pursue our hobby, it is to feel joy. Unfortunately, we sometimes confuse pleasure with lasting happiness. They are different. When we chase our momentary pleasure we often pay afterwards. The karma of a party is a hangover, the karma of overeating is feeling sick, the karma of spending too much time following my hobby is I haven't done my work or looked after my family.

Part of the yogic practice is in fact the ability to create space between my desire for pleasure (*raga*) and aversion to what I don't like (*dvesha*) so that we can discriminate and find the right path. The right path gives us pleasure in the long run; for example, practising to play the piano is dull and unexciting, but managing to play a piece is incredibly fulfilling and gives pleasure to so many people.

Yoga as a science of wellbeing

Yoga is a science of wellbeing, it works on every level of human existence to optimise our experience of life.

The physical practice ensures physical health and a strong immune system through its magical release of certain pressure points and so-called *nadis*.[1] The breathing practice ensures mental calm, and the meditation lends us insight into right action, delving deep into our intuition, to guide us forward through life. The philosophy in the ancient texts further gives concrete examples of tricky situations and lends us ideas on how to respond wisely. They open up vast secrets – sharing with us the beauty and depth of ancient and timeless wisdom on how to be a good human on this earth, thereby bringing meaning to our life.

As we spend time in meditation, we create a space, a pause for our minds, in order to recalibrate, to take the view from the top of the mountain on the vista of our life and ensure we are on the right path. This is why our teacher, Swami Vishnudevananda, said yoga was about the five points:

1. Proper exercise (asana)
2. Proper breathing (*pranayama* and conscious breathing)
3. Proper diet (vegetarian or conscious eating)
4. Proper relaxation (*savasana*)
5. Positive thinking and meditation (turning our thoughts around)

---

1 *Nadis* are similar but not equivalent to the Chinese meridians, that is, invisible energy lines that run throughout the whole body and are stimulated during asana.

Exercises and ideas for classes

I have always enjoyed the following story and use it many times to remind myself how to look at any given situation, and I often tell it to my students:

> Once upon a time there was a king who was very fond of hunting. He had a minister whose philosophy was that 'everything happens for the best'. No matter what, the minister infallibly said the same thing: 'Everything happens for the best!' This began to annoy the king. One day the king went out hunting. Somehow he fell off his horse and injured himself. His thumb had to be amputated. The king was very upset and despondent over the matter because it meant that he would not be able to hunt. As usual, the wise minister declared: 'Everything happens for the best!' The king was furious and retorted: 'What if I say you have lost your job?'; and then sent the minister away from the palace. The minister just said: 'Everything happens for the best!'
>
> Some time later the king again went out hunting. This time he managed to get himself lost in the forest and was kidnapped by a group of forest dwellers who were looking for a human to sacrifice to the goddess Kali! During the preparation they discovered with disgust that one of his thumbs was missing. Assuming that he had already been offered to the goddess and not wanting to make a second hand offering to Kali, they released him and sent him away. The king realised with relief: 'Indeed, everything happens for the best!' When he returned to the palace, he called his minister back and promoted him.

A question for your students: Can you think of times when you thought everything was going wrong in your life and afterwards you realise it was actually for the best?

Presence as joy

My teacher asked us: 'When was the moment you were the happiest?'

We all recounted endless stories of playing when we were little, doing something that excited us or that was difficult but satisfying. We were all describing the 'flow state'.

Psychologists Martin Seligman and Mihaly Csikszentmihalyi spoke of this state with some clarity as the basis of what they called the positive psychology movement.

The flow state has certain elements to it:

- *Clarity of goals and immediate feedback on progress.* For example, in a competition you know what you've got to achieve and you know exactly how well you are doing: whether you are winning or losing.
- *Complete concentration* on what one is doing at the present moment, with no room in the mind for any other information.
- *Actions and awareness are merged.* A guitar player merges with the instrument and becomes the music that he plays. The activity becomes almost automatic, and the involvement seems almost effortless (though far from being so in reality).
- *Losing awareness of oneself or self-consciousness* is also a common experience but, interestingly, after each flow experience the sense of self is strengthened and a person becomes more than he or she was before.
- *Sense of control* over what one is doing, with no worries about failure.
- *Transformation of time.* Usually, time passes much faster than expected. However, the reverse can also be true.
- *Activities are intrinsically rewarding.* We do the activity because we enjoy it, not because we are expecting rewards. (http://positivepsychology.org.uk/living-in-flow)

In a good yoga class we experience all or some of these elements, and they form an intrinsic part of why we keep coming back to the practice.

Thich Nhat Hanh is one of the most influential mindfulness practitioners today in the West and often speaks of the importance of being present. He speaks of the breath as the key to presence. Without awareness of breath, we cannot be present – it is our root into the present moment. Anchoring into our breath, we can bring ourselves back away from rumination, from anxiety or from fear.[2]

Try for yourself – the difficulty is remembering to practise when we are fearful or anxious. Keeping the intention for inner peace is a powerful tool indeed and ensures that you spread peace and understanding wherever you go.

When we allow ourselves to be completely present with our friends, they feel seen and heard, they feel loved. When we are not present it is often because we find the present moment too painful – whether it is because it is triggering uncomfortable feelings or whether it is because we are too preoccupied with thoughts (rumination); this makes us unhappy.

Bringing awareness to the pain and suffering is a particular mindfulness practice, which I find very important and useful and something we can all do.

The meditation goes like this:

> I see you suffering, I soothe your anger/grief/confusion – I am sorry you feel this way, anger/grief/suffering, I recognise you, you have been here before and I welcome you in as I soothe you. I sit with you calmly.

When we do this meditation sincerely, you will notice that the act of sitting with something helps to soothe and calm the emotions. They no longer come knocking on our door incessantly to be let in. They will leave the room after a while.

Gratitude exercise

Another wonderful and simple practice which I have done with my teens at home and in schools is the gratitude exercise. This involves a gratitude jar, in which we place notes of what we are grateful for. The simpler, the better – so it can be phrases such as the rain on the garden, riding my bike in the sun, eating apple pie. At the end you can take them out and study them, which makes you doubly happy! This is something you might like to do in your class.

2 Thich Nhat Hanh has written many books about the practice of breath meditation, such as *Planting Seeds: Practising Mindfulness with Children* (2011), but every one is a gem.

The other practice is before you go to bed at night you can list all the things you are grateful for. Have a little book by your bed and write in it every night.

Opposite thoughts exercise

Swami Sivananda, one of the great teachers of yoga philosophy, wrote 300 books, of which *Thought Power* (2009) is one of the most lucid.[3] In this book he describes how to overcome negative or unhelpful thought processes. He writes that we need to cultivate opposite thoughts. If we are feeling afraid of someone or something, we need to imagine with all our might how it might be to feel courageous. If we feel weak, we imagine the feeling of power and strength. I have found this works well, especially if we have a habitual thought or emotional pattern which is holding us back.

We need to be careful, though, that we do not use this as a way to suppress or repress feelings such as anger or grief.

Surrender

One of the most powerful tools that I learnt at the ashram was the concept of surrender. When we spend our lives resisting what is happening to us by wishing it was another way, we are wishing our life away and we are not trusting in the sanctity of life and the lessons that life has to offer us. Resistance is futile in most circumstances, whether it's going to school, getting up in the morning or going to work. Knowing when to surrender and when to fight is a wisdom in itself. We spend a great deal of our energy resisting the flow of life, leaving us precious little for when we need it. Flowing with what is and has to be is a deep wisdom.

However, it is not wise to surrender to all situations – if we see someone being beaten up and we are at their side, we do not surrender to the beating but we surrender instead to our obvious karma at that moment, which is to intervene.

There is a story which I think illustrates this perfectly:

---

3 Sivananda 2009.

A woman is shipwrecked far out at sea; all the other sailors drown. She swims aimlessly. She tells herself, 'God will protect me – I surrender to the situation, whatever will be will be.' A ship comes by, but she doesn't wave or do anything, she thinks I surrender, God will protect me; the ship passes by. She carries on praying, 'God save me, I surrender to your will'; a small rowing boat passes by and sees her – begs her to climb aboard – but she refuses, saying 'I surrender to God's wish, he will save me'; the rowing boat gives up and rows on. Finally a rescue helicopter comes past and drops down a ladder to her, begging her to grab it and step up, saying 'we are here to save you.' She refuses, saying 'God is going to save me, I surrender to his will.' They have to give up finally and fly away. After a gruesome night, she finally expires and slowly drowns. Her spirit goes to heaven. Perplexed, she turns to God and says: 'Why didn't you save me?' God answers: 'I tried three times, in the ship, the boat and the helicopter, but you refused.'

In that moment she realised that God was in everyone.

Practical exercises

Notice resistance and surrender in our practice. In Michael Lee's *Phoenix Rising* yoga therapy model,[4] there is a beautiful methodology of using the asanas and breathwork to become more aware of resistance and flow in the body.

I suggest you use this work to bring about peace of mind and to shift mood.

Script

- In *tadasana*,[5] feel into the left side of the body – are there any areas of tension or blockages, is there a flow anywhere or is there a specific pain anywhere along the left side? (Same for the right side.)
- Coming into forward bend, notice if there are any specific images, feelings, emotions or sensations that come up for

4 Lee 1997.

5 Mountain pose – when we stand at the front of our mat at the beginning of practice.

you in this posture. Where are they in the body? (Answers are internal.)

- And so on…use each asana to explore sensations, emotions, feelings and images or words that come up for the student. They might like to journal every so often.
- Then use the breath to clear the mind. Try not to overanalyse or work out what it all means, just observe, getting to know stuff that we sometimes ignore. In this way we learn to become much more present with ourselves. When this happens we can be more present with others and therefore come into the flow and be happy.
- You could use the opposite game here too, so when someone is feeling weak or fragile, after having felt into that, imagine how it might feel to be strong or courageous. Bring to mind an image of yourself as courageous; what would you do, how would you stand, how would you think?
- Flow state awareness: Bring them into a state where they are pushed to their limits physically without damaging themselves, but still within their comfort zone – where they can't think of anything else but what they are doing. You need to be very aware of each individual's capacity and sensitively design the class to their optimal state. Introduce them to the concept of flow state and ask them if there is anything else they do which brings them into this state.

Mindfulness exercise

Become present in the moment, noticing mind wandering and bringing it back to the present moment and the breath: *'I am breathing out, I spread love to every person I meet – I am breathing in, I welcome peace into my heart.'*

This might be a nice segue into meditation but let that happen naturally and wait for the teens to be ready for it. You will notice that, because of their youth, eagerness, suffering and natural curiosity, they will be keen to learn new things and get into them very quickly. However, meditation needs to be taught when they are completely ready, when they naturally come into stillness at the end of a yoga class and spontaneously want to stay in that state of bliss. Only teachers and therapists who practise meditation can teach it.

Pranayama

Breath of joy is effective and fun – standing in a wide stance, inhale your arms up and exhale your arms down, while bending your legs. On your exhalation, make a sighing sound. Repeat for a few minutes for full benefit.

Lion's breath

Kneeling, clench all your body, particularly the face; as you inhale and as you exhale, release your fists, with your tongue out of your mouth and eyes wide, as you look up at the ceiling – do this several times.

Asana

Come into a strong flowing practice that engages our awareness to start with and then come to slow awareness with the breath, watching thoughts and practising not identifying with them during postures.

It might be useful to use music to keep their attention in the classroom. (Your main aim as a teacher and therapist in this situation is to keep the mind from wandering.)

End with a long *savasana*, on the back for full effect of joy!

— Chapter 20 —

SERENITY

For your journal

Do you ever feel at peace?

If so, what makes you feel at peace?

What impact does it have on others?

Do you know how to use yogic techniques to reach peace?

What just happened? I opened my eyes. I was in the same room, but it seemed brighter, more beautiful. I felt like I had sat there for just a second or maybe a lifetime, who knew, but everything changed. I was calm, deep into my soul. I knew exactly what I had to do, how I had to act. I knew my path. My heart felt expanded and my mind felt still – I felt deeply peaceful, maybe for the first time. (Student on her experience of meditation)

What is serenity?

Peace of mind is happiness, health is wealth, yoga shows the way.

Swami Vishnudevananda

My teacher, Swami Vishnudevananda, introduced yoga to the West with this axiom, emblazoned in our minds. If peace of mind really is happiness, then we need to know how to achieve it. This book has gone some way to explaining how this works.

In Swami Venkatesananda's rendition and translation of *Vasistha's Yoga*,[1] considered by some to be one of the ancient texts of Yoga Vedanta philosophy, with some beautifully poetic and helpful dialogues that we can use to help us understand, there is one quote I particularly like:

> Parigha says: Oh king, all actions that are performed by one who is firmly established in equanimity are productive of joy, not those done by others. Are you established in that state of supreme peace in which no thoughts or notions arise in your mind, and which is known as Samadhi? (v 62, 63)...
>
> SURAGHU responds there is nothing that is worth desiring or renouncing. For as long as these things are seen as objects, they are nothing but concepts. When nothing is worth acquiring, it follows that nothing is worth renouncing. Good and evil, great and small, worthy or unworthy are all based on the notion of desirability. When desirability has no meaning, the others do not arise at all. There is truly no essence in all that is seen in the world – the mountains, the oceans, the forests, the men and women and all the objects. Hence there is no desire for them. When there is no desire, there is supreme peace at heart.

The notion that desire is at the heart of suffering is prevalent in all of Buddhism and permeates through yogic teachings too. It is a simple concept, although anathema to present values. The notion that desire is undesirable (!) works completely when we believe that everything is connected, spirit is in everything and we are all expressions of spirit – when we believe that life itself is a play of inter-related energies simply bouncing off each other, karma kicking off another karmic event and so on. We are simply the ball being bounced from one end to the other in the court of life. The choices we have are limited and come down to attitude: *How do I relate to what is happening to me? How can I change this situation? If I can't change it, how can I make the best of it?*

When we come into a situation where we feel immediately accepted and loved, where we feel compassion and empathy from the other beings in the room, we feel our heart expand and relax. Many people are attracted to this way of being and want to be like

1 Venkatesananda 1993.

this; they want to emanate joy, peace, love and acceptance, but too many fear-based emotions are in the way. These emotions contract us and make us smaller than who we are.

This experience of pain sometimes starts a journey in people. They have a burning desire to be free of pain, of the negative emotions, that pull them down.

There is a short, sweet story about that:

> *Once upon a time, there was a little old lady who lived on her own in a small and dark cottage in the woods. She was pretty content, but a simple woman. Every day she went about her business, collecting firewood, pulling the vegetables and cleaning her house. She sewed all her own clothes and the clothes of her friends and family too by hand, as it was in the olden days. One day in the height of summer, a friend came by to visit for a cup of tea and noticed that the old lady was distressed, looking here and there in the dirt and flower beds outside her cottage.*
>
> *'Dear friend, what are you looking for?'*
>
> *'I am looking for my needle.'*
>
> *Her friend joined her, looking here and there. After a while, things were looking hopeless, and her friend asked her: 'But where did you drop it?'*
>
> *'Oh, I dropped it in the house.'*
>
> *'But why are we looking for it here then?' exclaimed the friend.*
>
> *'Because it is light here,' says the woman.*

It is so common that we displace our need for tenderness and loving into consumption and absenteeism in relationship. When we feel pain because our needs are not met, we look outside, we look to blame another or to find another to fill the hole we experience inside, rather than looking inside for the light, the love and the tenderness. How many times have I sat in meditation and felt the angry, grabbing needs just melt away into a wholeness that I had forgotten through the busy, mindless day?

Famous psychologist Carl Jung once said:

> I have frequently seen people become neurotic when they content themselves with inadequate or wrong answers to the questions of life. They seek position, marriage, reputation, outward success of money, and remain unhappy and neurotic even when they have

> attained what they were seeking. Such people are usually confined within too narrow a spiritual horizon. Their life has not sufficient content, sufficient meaning. If they are enabled to develop into more spacious personalities, the neurosis generally disappears.[2]

Young people learn to conform to social norms and there are not many scenarios where the child is opened up to broad spiritual horizons, such as the ones that Jung mentions. So, how then, as Jung suggests, do we help young people expand into more spacious personalities? How do we bring them into a broader horizon?

In my opinion he is pointing towards religion as unsatisfactory. Religions have developed over millennia to satisfy the need in us for another dimension beyond the physical but we have moved into a new era where they are no longer enough. We are looking for a broader and more meaningful matrix, where we are not worshipping the God who had the experience (Jesus) but looking for the experience ourselves. We are no longer satisfied with the patriarchy of church where we are told what to believe and how to interpret someone else's experience but are looking for a direct experience that expands our view of the world around us and leads us to a visceral and unassailable truth. This truth can be experienced in meditation and long-term expert tuition of yoga, where the body is a vehicle for the spiritual experience.

Then the theory of yoga, written again and again in so many books, handed down generation to generation in the oral tradition, is no longer needed, as it is visceral. The experience of being at one with everyone and everything around becomes a daily habit. It needs to be cultivated by conscious awareness. At every moment, we need to remember that we are all made of energy, the same energy, and that we are in constant interaction with everything around us; the water, the earth, the air is entering and leaving our body at every second. We are permeable, we cannot shut out exterior influences. The follow-on from this experience is that we naturally respect everything around us, every living thing, every blade of grass and every drop of water. Our environment is literally an extension of us.

Rather than become sanctimonious and judgemental from this position, we become humble as we know that we have been or

2 Jung 1964, p.70.

could be every other person on this planet in this life or a past life; we are all just taking each other home. We are teachers for each other, who, hand in hand, guide and lead towards our ultimate goal, which is peace within ourselves and on our planet. This is not a new idea, nor is it an idea that is completely unique to yoga, it is universal, it binds all religions together.

The word Islam derives from the word meaning peace; in the Qu'ran it says:

> O You who believe! Enter absolutely into peace (Islam). (2, 208)

The Hebrew word for peace, *SHALOM*, comes from a root meaning 'completeness' and 'perfection'. So, when there is peace in Jewish terms, that means things are perfect: there is calm, security, prosperity and a general feeling of physical and spiritual wellbeing.

In the Bible, Colossians 3:15, it is written:

> Let the peace of Christ rule in your hearts, since as members of one body you were called to peace. And be thankful.

Truly then we all long for peace, it is our goal and our focus. Let yoga become a path to true inner peace for you and your student.

If you, as a teacher or therapist, are able to model a healthy and complete yoga practice, including finding peace within yourself, this will be the biggest teaching your students and clients will take away from you, both young and old. Imagine the impact your self-practice could have on young people and how, in turn, this could literally change the trajectory of the world, towards a more compassionate, conscious and caring community with peace at the core of every individual.

Asana exercises

(Ideally two hours when the students are proficient in asana and *pranayama*, when you know that they are able to witness the mind and come to a relatively peaceful place in their practice.)

Starting with a warm up, varied asanas that go through three chakras, from bottom to top; here is an example, but you can exchange the asanas to suit the class:

- Sun salutation.

- Mountain pose with deep breathing.
- Chair (focus on grounding through the legs and feet).
- Warrior two – focus on grounding, earth, everything that is solid in your body, how rooted you feel right now, the red colour bathes the body.
- Revolved warrior.
- Twist in warrior.
- Butterfly posture – focus on creativity, hips, water, everything that is fluid in you; *what do I really enjoy in life?* Colour orange bathes the body.
- Coming down on the back, coming into moving bridge, bringing awareness to the solar plexus, the power centre, the fire of change, the furnace of power – *in which areas of my life do I feel in control?* Colour yellow bathes my body.
- Coming into fish, opening the heart, bringing awareness to the heart, lifting and opening the area, air coming and going in the lungs, bathing in a green light, as we ask ourselves, *where is there compassion in my life?*
- Shoulder stand – awareness at the throat – colour blue, *I am listening and am heard*, ether[3] – the space between the skin and the muscle, between the muscle and the bone, space in the nerves, in the channels of the body.
- *Savasana*.
- Kneeling, with forehead on the floor, roll the head from right to left, massaging the head against the floor, bringing awareness to the forehead and the sixth chakra, between the eyebrows – bathing myself in a turquoise light, I ask myself *what is my path in life, what is the next step?* I trust my inner guidance.
- Coming into the hare posture, exactly the same, but rolling the head to and fro instead of side to side, massaging the

3 Ether in this context means the space between the bones, the space between the atoms, the space beyond air in the universe.

crown of the head, imagining a white light emanating from the crown of the head, sensing my belonging to the entire universe and everyone in the room. *I belong here and now.*

- *Savasana*.
- *Pranayama* – alternate nostril breath (5 minutes minimum).
- Chakra meditation exercises (as below).

Chakra meditation exercises

Base chakra – survival, connection with the earth, being grounded, safety, basic human needs

Sense: smell

Element: earth

Colour: red

Bija mantra:[4] lam

Question: Do I feel safe and secure?

Affirmation: I have everything I need (notice how this statement makes you feel)

Navel chakra – sexuality, sensuality, creativity, passion, vitality

Sense: taste

Element: water

Colour: orange

Bija mantra: vam

Question: Am I enjoying my life?

Affirmation: I feel safe and secure (notice how this makes you feel)

4 *Bija* mantra means 'seed mantra' and is the one-syllable sound that when said aloud activates the energy of the chakra.

Solar plexus chakra – identity, confidence, personality, power, spontaneous action, inner growth, warmth

Sense: sight

Element: fire

Colour: yellow

Bija mantra: ram

Question: Do I feel I am in control of my life?

Affirmation: I act with confidence and conviction (notice how this makes you feel)

Heart chakra – emotional centre, love, compassion, *agape*, understanding, forgiveness, centre of body, healer, loving ourselves, foundation of happiness and health

Sense: touch

Element: air

Colour: green

Bija mantra: yum

Question: Am I surrounded with love and able to receive and give love in equal measure?

Affirmation: I love myself and others unconditionally (notice how this makes you feel)

Throat chakra – sounds, communication, expression, truth, honesty, listening

Sense: hearing

Element: ether

Colour: blue

Bija mantra: hum

Question: Do I express my needs and feelings accurately and eloquently?

Affirmation: I speak my truth and am heard (notice how that makes you feel)

Eyebrow chakra – intuition, insight; when this is blocked there is self-doubt and mistrust

Colour: turquoise

Bija mantra: om

Question: Am I sure of my path and what I have to offer the world?

Affirmation: I see clearly what is (notice how this makes you feel)

Crown chakra – connection with the divine, one-ness, thousand petal lotus, positive thought patterns, inspiration for spiritual wellbeing, channels life energy into our system, aligns and balances all chakras – bathed in purple light, sacred wisdom

Colour: white/purple

Bija mantra: the sound of silence

Question: Do I feel a connection with the divine?

Affirmation: I know the truth (notice how this makes you feel)

Mantra or breath meditation – sitting or lying for 15–30 minutes, depending on group, watching the body, watching the breath and watching the thoughts, sensations and feelings.

— Chapter 21 —

CONCLUSION

You do not need to seek freedom in a different land, for it exists in your own body, mind and soul.

B. K. S. Iyengar[1]

The impetus for this book was the undisputable fact that young people are struggling with mental health problems to an unacceptable degree and that yoga may be a modality which addresses most of the problems exhibited today among this population. With this in mind, I have, in these pages, outlined the social, physical, mental and spiritual development and needs of the teen today and then drawn on the wisdom of the vast science of yoga to support optimal development. I hope your understanding of yoga and teens has broadened and deepened. The questions, the science, the suggestions and the exercises are aimed at bringing you and the teen to a higher level of awareness of what it means to be resilient, happy, successful and free.

I have briefly touched on some of the most prevalent issues that we come across in the field of adolescents today. You might well find some of the practices and skills that you have learned are transferable to other conditions. Many of the exercises suggested for teens struggling with anxiety would also apply to those who struggle with chronic stress. Similarly, some of the exercises for depression might well suit those who have suffered bereavement. PTSD and trauma are common among certain populations and could benefit from some of the exercises in the anxiety chapter.

Step by step, I have taken you through each 'layer' of the teen, the physical body, the breath, the mind, the wisdom and, finally,

1 Iyengar 2008, p.22.

taking them to their very own bliss. That is not dependent on anyone but ourselves and ultimately needs no effort; once the groundwork is laid, it is always there, at the centre of our being, and as long as we practise we will have glimpses of this state which soon becomes the ground state, the default setting. As Dan Siegel says so eloquently, your mind state becomes your mind trait; in other words, what we practise is who we become.[2]

We have taken a look at only some of the many and various techniques that have been taught and handed down through the millennia to gain calm, truth, insight, joy and enlightenment (*sat-chid-ananda*). Together we have tracked in detail how yoga works to ensure homeostasis – balance – in everyday life. Neuroscience is a young science, and most researchers in the field accept that they know very little and that we are only starting to understand how the brain works. I am excited to be sharing cutting-edge research with you and look forward to getting even more clarity on brain function and yoga as the research unfolds.

Yoga as relaxation

When we learn to relax completely into our lives, releasing tension in our relationships, in our bodies, in our minds and in our hearts, we let go of drama and conflict, we surrender and find freedom from outside pressures of all kinds. Our experience of life becomes subtler, more careful, more compassionate. With the help of yoga I believe that we can move from anxiety towards radical self-care, from radical self-care to becoming an engaged citizen, and then onwards to become warriors of peace, especially if we start yoga at a young age, before many habits have taken root.

Technology of wellbeing

Yoga is a *technology of wellbeing*. A technology is a set of various techniques that will have the same result every time, which is the case with yoga. We know that if we do a certain sequence or a certain breathing technique, we will come out feeling a certain way; if we move our body a little, it will release tension or make us

2 Video interview with author, 6 June 2016.

stronger; if we move our mind a little, it will support a healthier outlook on life. If we move our ego a little, we can get out of our own way!

When we share yoga with young people, it is my experience that they are less likely to fall sick and more likely to stay happy and reach their goals. The yoga will bring them clarity of mind, courage and compassion. The power of yoga over singular modalities like mindfulness or meditation is that it is a step-ladder approach, offering something to everyone. It is a catch-all technique which builds from values, to postures, to breathing, and then on to mindfulness and finally meditation.

In this way, step by step, yoga takes us beyond happiness to serenity. To be in the moment, to notice the preciousness of the life we are living, we need to learn how to drop anxiety and worry and to serve others. We need to embody this and thereby share with others how to let go and enjoy the ride, without trying to control it.

> A student came into my class one day and told me that the biology teacher meditated. I asked: 'How do you know – did she do it in class with you?' He shook his head and said: 'No, I can tell.' 'How can you tell?' I asked. 'The way she is, she is calm, kind and never raises her voice!' 'How was the lesson?' I asked. 'Much better,' he said, smiling, 'everyone was focused and calm.' 'Did she teach you any meditation?' 'No, she didn't have to.'

The student benefited, as did the entire classroom, from the teacher's practice, and she didn't even share it openly.

Meaning of yoga

Yoga means union, the union between body, mind and spirit, the union between you and other people, the union or connection between you and Nature and the whole of the living universe. Therefore, the practice of yoga is practising connecting with ourselves and with others. When we connect and feel the union with Nature and others, we expand into a higher awareness, as if we are looking from a high platform. With this dual form of attention, that of 'me' and that of 'us', we learn to look at what is preventing that connection, what is isolating us and dividing us, what is causing imbalance and dis-ease, and we learn to compassionately dissolve those elements: the need to be right, the desire to control, the desire for power over others and the critical voice that we direct towards ourselves. Because suffering comes from wanting things to be different from what they are, from resisting what is. When we believe that the universe is good and we learn to view everyone and everything with an unconditional positive regard, then we are more able to trust that all will be well. When we are able to divorce ourselves from our little story, witnessing our thoughts, we can place ourselves in a more realistic context, as one star of many in the heavens, as one piece of the jigsaw, not the central piece but an important piece. With this insight we become humble, courageous, resilient and of service to others and the greater good. Moreover, our emotions no longer wreak havoc over our lives, as we favour the calm over the drama. This meta-cognition saves us from anxiety and fear, by seeing our role in the bigger picture. You now have a four-dimensional map to teens, combined I hope with the complete conviction that at the heart of them lies bliss, joy, beauty and truth, as at the heart of every living creature. These qualities are the qualities of being-ness.

Yoga as service

When I told my teacher that I was writing this book he reminded me that one of the main tenets of yoga is to serve others and, also, that yoga was offered for free historically. It should be taught, he says, in the way a mother teaches her child, in the spirit of service, a free life lesson, which will help young people make sense of their life, care for themselves intelligently and be of service to others and their community. In our society, to work for free is mostly impossible and in some cases would undermine the work we do. However, I encourage you to offer free classes on occasion to those who need it and possibly also to school teachers now and again, so that they too can enjoy the benefits of yoga and pass that on to their students. When we share yoga with those who work with young people on a daily basis, then the practices will filter into their everyday lives and start to really facilitate change. Also, I hope that the young people you teach will go on to share the secrets of yoga with their peers to help and support them in times of need and distress.

The future is bright

The future is bright for teen yoga across the world. Sport England has been supporting yoga classes and training courses for the past ten years, investing around half a million pounds altogether in yoga as a tool to activate those who have no interest in sport. As I write, we are rolling out yoga for disadvantaged students across Europe in five different contexts to 750 young people and their teachers or youth leaders. Historically I have found this holistic (student and teacher) approach to be the most successful, as when the leaders incorporate the techniques in daily life it is more likely to be accepted and adopted by the teens themselves too. We are also currently measuring the impact of yoga on the general teen population across the UK, reaching around 1000 teens, together with Westminster University's Psychology Department. The results of this project will be published and will form one of the biggest studies ever done of this age group, potentially impacting on government initiatives for wellbeing both in the UK and abroad.

Many of my students have grasped the power that yoga can have in changing the trajectory of our future. I am particularly warmed by the initiatives of the small group of women in Abu Dhabi who see yoga as a way to pacify Islamic extremists and to curb radicalisation among young men and women there. My annual trips to the United Arab Emirates allow me to momentarily delve into the Muslim world of women. Behind the veil, I notice the impact that yoga is having in their lives, liberating and empowering them and deepening their relationship with Islam through the visceral experience of spirituality.

As I write I am preparing my first lecture to Postgraduate Certificate in Education (PGCE) students at a university in the UK, on how to incorporate yoga in the classroom, making these teachers the first ones to be intrinsically trained in yoga. The UK government is taking steps to incorporate yoga in society, with the formation of the All Party Parliamentary Group for Yoga in Society in 2018, with yoga in schools being one of four verticals, also including yoga in prisons, yoga in the workplace and yoga in healthcare. The openness to and interest in yoga within Westminster is supported by the success of the mindfulness initiatives, started in exactly the same manner several years ago.

Teachers are leaders, they drive the future. They influence hundreds of future leaders every day with their manner, their ideas and their teaching. If you are sharing life skills with young people, you are part of determining the future of our planet. If you have the skill of teaching and sharing and are sharing yoga with young people, the world has a brighter future, brimming with a positive outlook, peace and compassion.

More funding and more research is needed to evaluate and support initiatives that are happening on grassroots levels with passionate individuals like yourself, who have a single vision, that of alleviating suffering among the young in order to ensure a peaceful and sustainable future for us and our planet.

My intention has always been to empower young people, so it seems only fit to end this book with a quote from one of my most mischievous and vital 11-year-old boys who came to yoga every week for three years until he was forced to leave as he was too old for the group; I love the way he describes his experience of yoga:

> The main thing it's about is just you, like yoga's different for every person, it's for you, it's not the main purpose of football [which] is about getting the ball in the goal, because there's...nothing to really help you, it's just your own body, so it's your limit to your strength, that's the main point of yoga...
>
> Like your limit's like something that I can't yet do, like I can't do a handstand or a bridge, so I can just build up to that by strengthening all my muscles, so I'm pushing my limits further and further...
>
> It just makes me feel happier and it makes me remember who I am sometimes because sometimes you're so caught up in school, then you forget who you really are sometimes, like you're in the school uniform, you have all the books in your bag that you've written in, but then you just run around places, you're not in your own body but you are, and in yoga after school or in the middle of school you can just relax and breakdown ...

Bibliography

Alberti, G., Zimmet, P., Shaw, J., Bloomgarden, Z. *et al.* (2004) 'Type 2 diabetes in the young: The evolving epidemic. The International Diabetes Federation Consensus Workshop.' *Diabetes Care 27*, 7, 1798–1811.

American College of Pediatricians (2016) 'The impact of pornography on children.' American College of Pediatricians. Accessed on 18/03/2018 at www.acpeds.org/the-college-speaks/position-statements/the-impact-of-pornography-on-children.

Bainbridge, E. (2017) Interview, Instill Conference, 11 November (Interviewer R. Watkins-Davis).

Begley, S. (2007) *Train Your Mind, Change Your Brain.* New York: Ballantine Books.

Biddulph, S. (2013) *Raising Girls.* New York: Harper.

Biddulph, S. (2015) *Raising Boys: Why Boys Are Different and How to Help Them Become Happy and Well-Balanced Men.* New York: Harper Thorsons.

Biddulph, S. (2015) *The Complete Secrets of Happy Children.* New York: Harper Thorsons.

Blakemore, D. S. (2015) Interview, *The Life Scientific*, 25 March (Interviewer J. Al-Khalili).

Bowlby, J. (1969) *Attachment and Loss, Volume 1.* New York: Basic Books.

Bradford, E. (2018) 'Half of teenagers sleep deprived, say experts.' BBC, 26 August. Accessed on 16/03/2018 at www.bbc.co.uk/news/uk-scotland-23811690.

Brinkhues, S., Dukers-Muijrers, N., Hoebe, C. and van der Kallen, C. (2017) 'Socially isolated individuals are more prone to have newly diagnosed and prevalent type 2 diabetes mellitus – the Maastricht Study.' *BMC Public Health 17*, 995.

Brown, C. (2017) *The Modern Yoga Bible.* London: Godsfield Press.

Brunton, P. (1934) *A Search in Secret India.* New York: Harmony Books.

Butzer, B., Bury, D., Telles, S. and Khalsa, S. B. (2016) 'Implementing yoga within the school curriculum: A scientific rationale for improving social-emotional learning and positive student outcomes.' *Journal of Children's Services 11*, 1, 3–24.

Camus, A. (1942) *The Outsider.* London: Penguin Books.

Carrington, D. (2016) 'Three-quarters of UK children spend less time outdoors than prison inmates – survey.' *Guardian*, 25 March.

Cartwright, T. (2017) *Big Yoga Survey.* London: Westminster University. Unpublished.

Chopra, D. (2006) *Fire in the Heart: A Spiritual Guide for Teens.* New York: Simon & Schuster.

Connolly, A. (2016) *Health Survey for England 2015: Children's Body Mass Index, Overweight and Obesity.* London: National Statistics.

Covey, S. R. (2005) *The 8th Habit: From Effectiveness to Greatness.* London: Simon & Schuster.

Cross, F. (2017) Interview, Instill Conference, 11 November (Interviewer R. Watkins-Davis).

Delaney, B. (2017) 'The yoga industry is booming – but does it make you a different person?' *Guardian*, 17 September.

Department for Education (2014) 'Promoting fundamental British values as part of SMSC in schools: Departmental advice for maintained schools.' Accessed on 05/04/2018 at www.gov.uk/government/uploads/system/uploads/attachment_data/file/380595/SMSC_Guidance_Maintained_Schools.pdf.

Department of Health (2008) *Children and Young People in Mind: The Final Report of the National CAMHS Review.* London: Stationery Office.

Desikachar, T. (1999) *The Heart of Yoga: Developing a Personal Practice.* Rochester, VT: Inner Traditions/Bear and Company.

Desikachar, T. and Krusche, H. (2014) *Freud and Yoga: Two Philosophies of Mind Compared* (A. M. Hodges, Trans.). New York: North Point Press.

Devlin, M. J., Yanovski, S. Z. and Wilson, G. T. (2000) 'Obesity: What mental health professionals need to know.' *American Journal of Psychiatry 157*, 66, 854–866.

Dinsmore-Tuli, U. (2014) *Yoni Shakti: A Woman's Guide to Power and Freedom through Yoga and Tantra.* London: Yogawords.

Dion, R. (2017) Interview, Instill Conference, 11 November (Interviewer R. Watkins-Davis).

Durgananda, S. (2010) *Patanjali's Sutras.* New Delhi: Mangalam Books.

Euswaran, E. (2007) *The Bhagavad Gita.* Tomales, CA: Nilgiri Press.

Euswaran, E. (2007) *The Upanishads.* Tomales, CA: Nilgiri Press.

Feuerstein, G. (2001) *The Yoga Tradition: Its History, Literature, Philosophy and Practice.* New York: Hohm Press.

Forster, K. (2017) 'Third of NHS children's mental health services "face cuts or closure".' *Independent*, 22 May. Accessed on 16/03/2018 at www.independent.co.uk/news/health/nhs-children-mental-health-services-cuts-or-closure-third-downsizing-survey-staff-conservatives-a7749616.html.

Gambhirananda, S. (2010) *Mandukya Upanishad.* New Delhi, India: Advaita Ashrama.

Gangadhar, B. (2013) 'Cortisol and antidepressant effects of yoga.' *Indian Journal of Psychiatry* 55, 400–404.

Golding, W. (1954) *Lord of the Flies.* London: Faber and Faber.

Goleman, D. (2017) *The Science of Meditation.* London: Penguin Life.

Greenland, S. K. (2010) *The Mindful Child.* New York: Simon & Schuster.

Gruber, T. (2005) *Yoga Pretzels: 50 Fun Yoga Activities for Kids and Grownups.* Oxford: Barefoot Books.

Guardian (2011) 'Children's eating disorder figures cause alarm.' *Guardian*, 1 August.

Haas, S. (2015) *The Book of Dharma: Making Enlightened Choices.* Burgess Hill: Veda Wisdom Books.

Haas, S. (2018) *Yoga and the Dark Night of the Soul.* London: Veda Wisdom Books.

Hale, L. and Guan, S. (2015) 'Screen time and sleep among school-aged children and adolescents: A systematic literature review.' *Sleep Medicine Reviews*, 21, 50–58.

Hall, M., Baum, A., Buysse, D. J., Prigerson, H. G., Kupfer, D. J. and Reynolds, C. F. (1998) 'Sleep as a mediator of the stress-immune relationship.' *Psychosomatic Medicine 60*, 48–51.

Hanh, T. N. (2011) *Planting Seeds: Practising Mindfulness with Children.* Berkeley, CA: Parallax Press.

Harper, J. C. (2016) *Best Practice for Yoga in Schools.* Boston, MA: YSC Omega Publications.

Hughes, D. (2016) 'Illnesses associated with lifestyle cost the NHS £11bn.' BBC, 25 September. Accessed on 16/03/2018 at www.bbc.co.uk/news/health-37451773.

Isherwood, C. (1949) *Vedanta for the Western World.* London: Unwin Books.

Iyengar, B. (2008) *Light on Life: The Journey to Wholeness, Inner Peace and Ultimate Freedom.* London: Rodale.

Jenkins, R. (2017) 'Study: More recreational screen-time linked to worse mental health in teens.' *PsyPost*, 11 August. Accessed on 16/03/2018 at www.psypost.org/2017/08/study-recreational-screen-time-linked-worse-mental-health-teens-49470.

Jensen, F. (2015) *The Teenage Brain.* New York: HarperCollins.

Jeter, P. E., Slutsky, J., Singh, N. and Khalsa, S. B. (2015) 'Yoga as a therapeutic intervention: A bibliometric analysis of published research studies from 1967 to 2013.' *Journal of Alternative and Complementary Medicine 21*, 586–592.

Johari, H. (2000) *Chakras: Energy Centers of Transformation.* Merrimac, MA: Destiny.

Judith, A. (1987) *Wheels of Life: Users' Guide to the Chakra System.* Woodbury, MN: Llewellyn Publications.

Jung, C. (1964) *Civilization in Transition: Collected Works, Volume 10.* London: Routledge.

Kabat-Zinn, J. (2005) 'Mindful yoga, movement and meditation.' *Yoga Chicago*, April. Accessed on 16/03/2018 at http://yogachicago.com/2014/03/mindful-yoga-movement-and-meditation.

Kaminoff, L. (2011) *Yoga Anatomy.* Cambridge, MA: Human Kinetics.

Khalsa, S.B. (2016) *Yoga in Education.* Presentation, Instill Conference, 8–9 July.

Khalsa, S. B. and Butzer, B. (2016) 'Yoga in school settings: A research review.' *Annals of the New York Academy of Sciences 1373*, 1, 45–55.

Kleeman, J. (Reporter) and Drury, M. (Director) (2017) Sleepless Britain [Television series episode]. In O'Connor, A. and Kleeman, N. (Executive Producers), *Panorama*. London, UK: BBC.

Knoll, L. J., Magis-Weinberg, L., Speekenbrink, M. and Blakemore, S. J. (2015) 'Social Influence on Risk Perception During Adolescence. *Psychol Sci 26*, 5, 583–592.

Kolk, B. (2015) *The Body Keeps the Score.* London: Penguin.

Krishnananda, S. (2006) *Chandogya Upanishad.* Rishikesh: Divine Life Society.

Krushnakumar, D., Hamblin, M. R. and Lakshmanan, S. (2015) 'Meditation and yoga can modulate brain mechanisms that affect behaviour and anxiety – a modern scientific perspective.' *Ancient Science 2*, 1, 13–19.

Kumar, S. (2010) 'Need for determining the incidence and prevalence of JIA in developing countries: The Indian predicament.' *British Society for Rheumatology 49*, 1598–1599.

Lapsley, D. K., Rice, K. G. and FitzGerald, D. P. (1990) 'Adolescent attachment, identity, and adjustment to college: Implications for the continuity of adaptation hypothesis.' *Journal of Counseling and Development 68*, 5, 561–565.

Lee, M. (1997) *Phoenix Rising – A Bridge from Body to Soul.* New York: Health Communications.

Livingstone, S. (2002) *The Media Rich Home: Balancing Public and Private Lives.* London: Sage.

Long, R. (2009) *Key Muscles of Yoga: Your Guide to Functional Anatomy in Yoga.* Baldwinsville, NY: Bandha Yoga Publications.

Macleod, J., Oakes, R., Copello, A., Crome, I. *et al.* (2004) 'Psychological and social sequelae of cannabis and other illicit drug use by young people: A systematic review of longitudinal, general population studies.' *The Lancet 363*, 9421, 1579–1588.

Maehle, G. (2001) *Ashtanga Yoga: Practice and Philosophy.* Novato, CA: New World Library.

Maguire, E. A., Wollett, K. and Spiers, H. J. (2006) 'London Taxi Drivers and Bus Drivers: A Structural MRI and Neuropsychological Analysis.' *Hippocampus 16*, 12, 1091–1101.

Martin-Merino, E., Ruigomez, A., Wallander, M., Johansson, S. and Garcia Rodriguez, L. (2009) 'Prevalence, incidence, morbidity and treatment patterns in a cohort of patients diagnosed with anxiety in UK primary care.' *Family Practice 27*, 1, 9–16.

Matousek, M. (2012) *When You Are Falling, Dive.* London: Hay House.

Mcleod, S. (2007) 'Bowlby's attachment theory.' *Simply Psychology.* Accessed on 16/03/2018 at www.simplypsychology.org/bowlby.html.

Mojtabai, R., Olfson, M. and Han, B. (2016) 'National trends in the prevalence and treatment of depression in adolescents and young adults.' *Pediatrics 138*, 6.

Morgan, A. (2013) *How Young People Explain the Benefits of Yoga.* Leeds: Insitute of Psychological Sciences, University of Leeds.

Morgan, D. (2010) 'Mindfulness-based cognitive therapy for depression: A new approach to preventing relapse.' *Psychotherapy Research 13*, 1, 123–125.

Morgan, N. (2013) *Blame My Brain.* London: Walker Books.

Muktibodhananda, S. (2016) *Hatha Yoga Pradipika.* Munger: Yoga Publications Trust.

NHS Digital (n.d.) 'National Child Measurement Programme shows increased obesity prevalence in primary schools.' Accessed on 05/04/2018 at https://digital.nhs.uk/article/923/National-Child-Measurement-Programme-shows-increased-obesity-prevalence-in-primary-schools.

NSPCC (2018) 'Mental health and suicidal thoughts.' NSPCC. Accessed on 16/03/2018 at www.nspcc.org.uk/preventing-abuse/keeping-children-safe/mental-health-suicidal-thoughts-children.

Oakley, B. (2012) *Pathological Altruism.* Oxford: Oxford University Press.

Ogden, P. (2006) *Trauma and the Body: A Sensorimotor Approach to Psychotherapy.* New York: Norton Series on Interpersonal Neurobiology.

Orzech, K., Salafsky, D. B. and Hamilton, L. A. (2011) 'The state of sleep among college students at a large public university.' *Journal of American College Health 59*, 7, 612–619.

Osteopenia3 (2018) 'Young women with osteopenia.' Accessed on 18/03/2018 at www.osteopenia3.com/Young-women-with-Osteopenia.html.

Porges, S. (2001) 'The polyvagal theory: Phylogenetic substrates of a social nervous system.' *International Journal of Psychophysiology 42*, 2, 123–146.

Purperhart, H. (2007) *The Yoga Adventure for Children.* Alameda, CA: Hunter House.

Rama, S. (1999) *Yoga and Psychotherapy: The Evolution of Consciousness.* Honesdale, PA: Himalayan Institute Press.

Reyna, V. F. and Farley, F. (2015) 'Risk and rationality in adolescent decision-making: Implications for theory, practice, and public policy. *Psychological Science in the Public Interest 7*, 1, 1–44.

Robinson, O. J., Vytal, K., Cornwell, B. R. and Grillon, C. (2013) 'The impact of anxiety upon cognition: Perspectives from human threat of shock studies.' *Frontiers in Human Neuroscience 7*, 203.

Rodrigues, D. (2018) 'Hormone yoga therapy.' Accessed on 18/03/2018 at www.dinahrodrigues.com.br/home-en.

SAMHSA (2017) 'Prescription drug misuse and abuse.' Accessed on 18/03/2018 at www.samhsa.gov/topics/prescription-drug-misuse-abuse.

Saraswati, S. S. (2004) *Yoga Education for Children.* Bihar: Yoga Publications Trust.

Scaravelli, V. (1991) *Awakening the Spine: The Stress-Free Yoga That Works with the Body to Build Health, Vitality and Energy.* London: Pinter & Martin.

Scheel, J. (2018) 'Mothers, eating disorders and histories of trauma.' *Psychology Today.* Accessed on 18/03/2018 at www.psychologytoday.com/blog/when-food-is-family/201801/mothers-eating-disorders-and-histories-trauma.

Schiffman, E. (1997) *Yoga: The Spirit of Moving into Stillness.* New York: Simon & Schuster.

Selfharm UK (2018) 'Self-harm statistics.' Selfharm UK. Accessed on 18/03/2018 at www.selfharm.co.uk/get-information/the-facts/self-harm-statistics.

Sellgren, K. (2016) 'Pornography "desensitising young people".' BBC, 15 June. Accessed on 18/03/2018 at www.bbc.co.uk/news/education-36527681.

Siegel, D. D. (2011) 'The Healthy Mind Platter.' Accessed on 18/03/2018 at www.drdansiegel.com/resources/healthy_mind_platter/.

Siegel, D. J. (2013) *Brainstorm.* New York: Penguin, Putnam.

Singleton, M. (2010) *Yoga Body: The Origins of Modern Posture Practice.* London: Oxford University Press.

Sivananda, S. (2004) *Bliss Divine.* Rishikesh: Divine Life Society.

Sivananda, S. (2009) *Thought Power.* Rishikesh: Divine Life Society.

Sivananda Yoga Vedanta Centre (2000) *New Book of Yoga.* London: Sivananda Yoga Vedanta Centre.

Sivananda Yoga Vedanta Centre (2003) *Sivananda Companion to Meditation.* London: Sivananda Yoga Vedanta Centre.

Sivananda Yoga Vedanta Centre (2003) *Sivananda Companion to Yoga.* London: Sivananda Yoga Vedanta Centre.

Sivertsen, B., Lallukka, T., Salo, P., Pallesen, S. *et al.* (2014) 'Insomnia as a risk factor for ill health: Results from the large population-based prospective HUNT Study in Norway.' *Journal of Sleep Research 23*, 2, 121–123.

Stefan Schmidt, H. W. (2014) *Meditation – Neuroscientific Approaches and Philosophical Implications.* New York: Springer.

Streeter, C. C., Whitfield, T. H., Owen, L., Rein, T. *et al.* (2010) 'Effects of yoga versus walking on mood, anxiety and brain GABA levels: A randomized controlled MRS study.' *Journal of Alternative and Complementary Medicine 16*, 11, 1145–1152.

Styles, M. (2000) *Structural Yoga Therapy.* Newburyport, MA: Red Wheel.

Telles, S., Nilkhamal, S. and Balkrishna, A. (2012) 'Managing mental health disorders resulting from trauma through yoga.' *Depression Research and Treatment 2012*, 401–513.

Telles, S., Singh, N., Bhardwaj, A. K., Kumar, A. and Balkrishna, A. (2013) 'Effect of yoga or physical exercise on physical, cognitive and emotional measures in children: A randomized controlled trial.' *Child and Adolescent Psychiatry and Mental Health 7*, 37.

Torjesen, I. (2016) 'Use of antidepressants in children soars by 50% in the UK.' *Pharmaceutical Journal*, 11 March. Accessed on 18/03/2018 at www.pharmaceutical-journal.com/news-and-analysis/use-of-antidepressants-in-children-soars-by-50-in-the-uk/20200856.article.

Turkle, S. (2012) *Alone Together: Why We Expect More from Technology and Less from Each Other.* New York: Basic Books.

Uebelacker, L. (2010) 'Hatha yoga for depression: Critical review of the evidence for efficacy, plausible mechanisms of action and directions for future research.' *Journal of Psychiatric Practice 16*, 1, 22–33.

Venkatesananda, S. (1993) *Vasistha's Yoga.* New York: State University of New York Press.

Vishnudevananda, S. (1961) *The Complete Illustrated Book of Yoga.* Delhi: Souvenir Publishers.

Vishnudevananda, S. (1978) *Meditation and Mantras.* London: Sivananda Yoga Vedanta Centre.

Waller, P. (2012) *Holistic Anatomy: An Integrative Guide to the Human Body.* Berkeley, CA: North Atlantic Books.

Watkins-Davis, R. (2017) Interview, Instill Conference, 11 November (Interviewer C. Martinus).

Watts, A. (2017) Interview, Instill Conference, 11 November (Interviewer R. Watkins-Davis).

Weston, P. (2017) 'Children's screen time rises from three hours a day in 2000 to nearly five hours (but experts insist technology is NOT taking over their lives).' *Daily Mail*, 21 December. Accessed on 18/03/2018 at www.dailymail.co.uk/sciencetech/article-5203377/Young-people-spend-FIVE-hours-day-looking-screen.html.

Wikipedia (2018) 'Maharishi School.' Accessed on 18/03/2018 at https://en.wikipedia.org/wiki/Maharishi_School_(UK).

Young, J. L. (2015) *Is Obesity a Mental Health Issue?* New York: Psychology Today.

YoungMinds (2018) 'Mental health statistics.' *YoungMinds*, 10 January. Accessed on 16/03/2018 at https://youngminds.org.uk/about-us/media-centre/mental-health-stats/?gclid=EAIaIQobChMInsva_tab2QIV6LftCh0OSgmkEAAYAiAAEgIVEfD_BwE.

Zosel, A., Bartelson, B. B., Bailey, E., Lowenstein, S. and Dart, R. (2013) 'Characterization of adolescent prescription drug abuse and misuse using the researched abuse diversion and addiction related surveillance system.' *Journal of the American Academy of Child and Adolescent Psychiatry 52*, 2, 196–204.

Index

If you enjoyed the book and would like to pursue this topic, please visit our website for upcoming courses around the world and online - www.teenyoga.com

You can also find us on:
Facebook – teenyogamindfulness
Instagram – teenyogafoundation
Twitter– TeenYogaGlobal

If you would like to get involved in our charity, please visit www.teenyogafoundation.com

Please contact the author with any queries at Charlotta@teenyoga.com